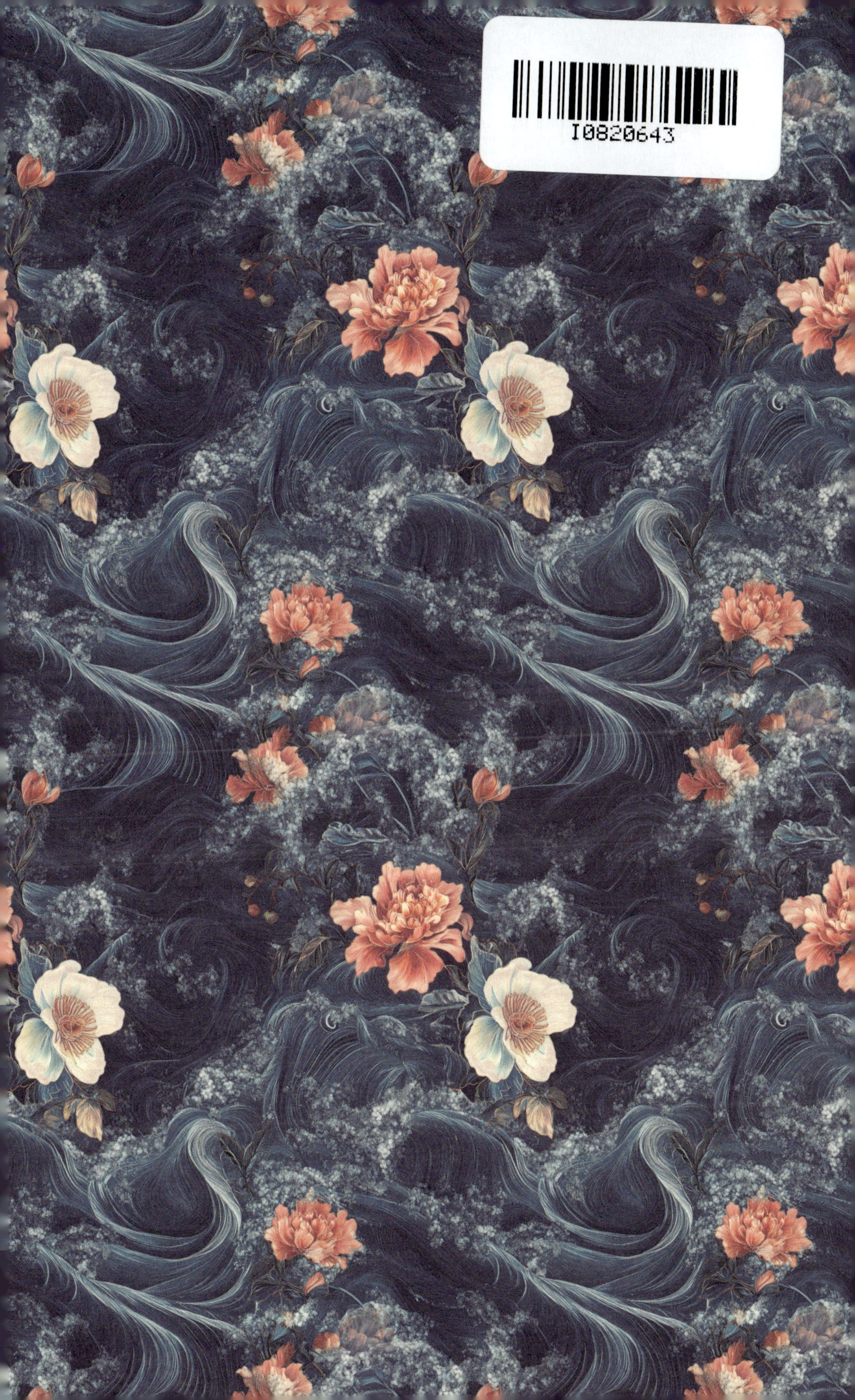
I0820643

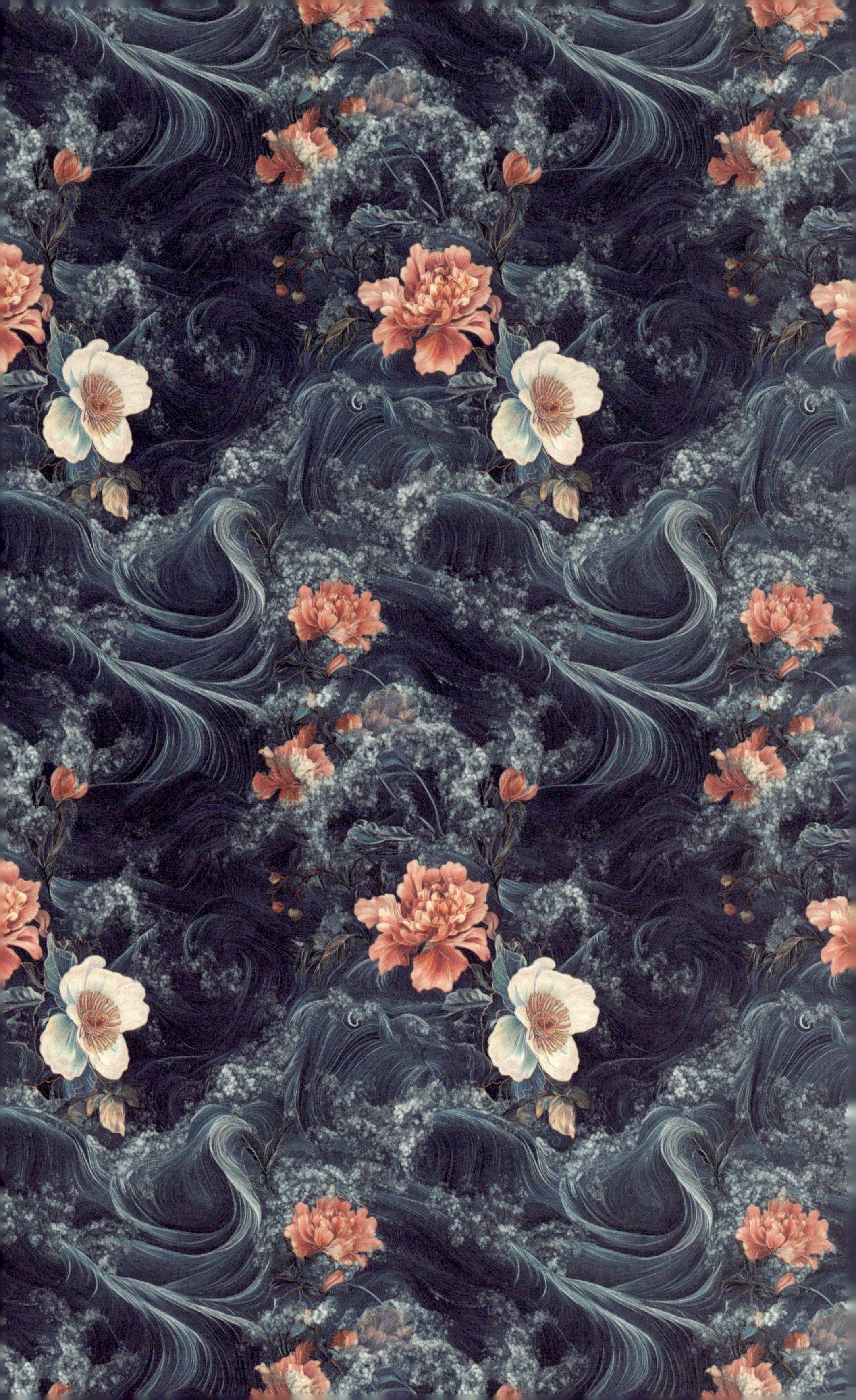

UNFIXED

A MEMOIR OF FAMILY, MYSTERY, AND THE CURRENTS THAT CARRY YOU HOME

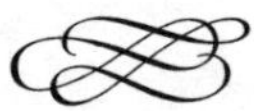

KIMBERLY WARNER

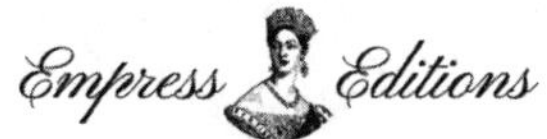

Empress Editions ~ No 2
Published by Empress Editions LLC
First Printing

Typeset in Baskerville in Cambridge.
Printed and bound in China by Cynthia.
ISBN 979-8-992386-547

Empress Editions
303 Third Street
Cambridge, MA 02142
+1 617.580.5266
empresseditions.io

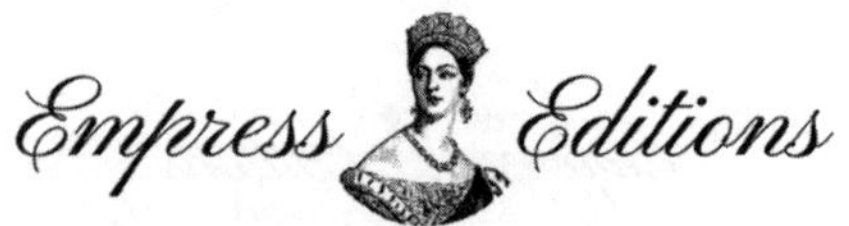

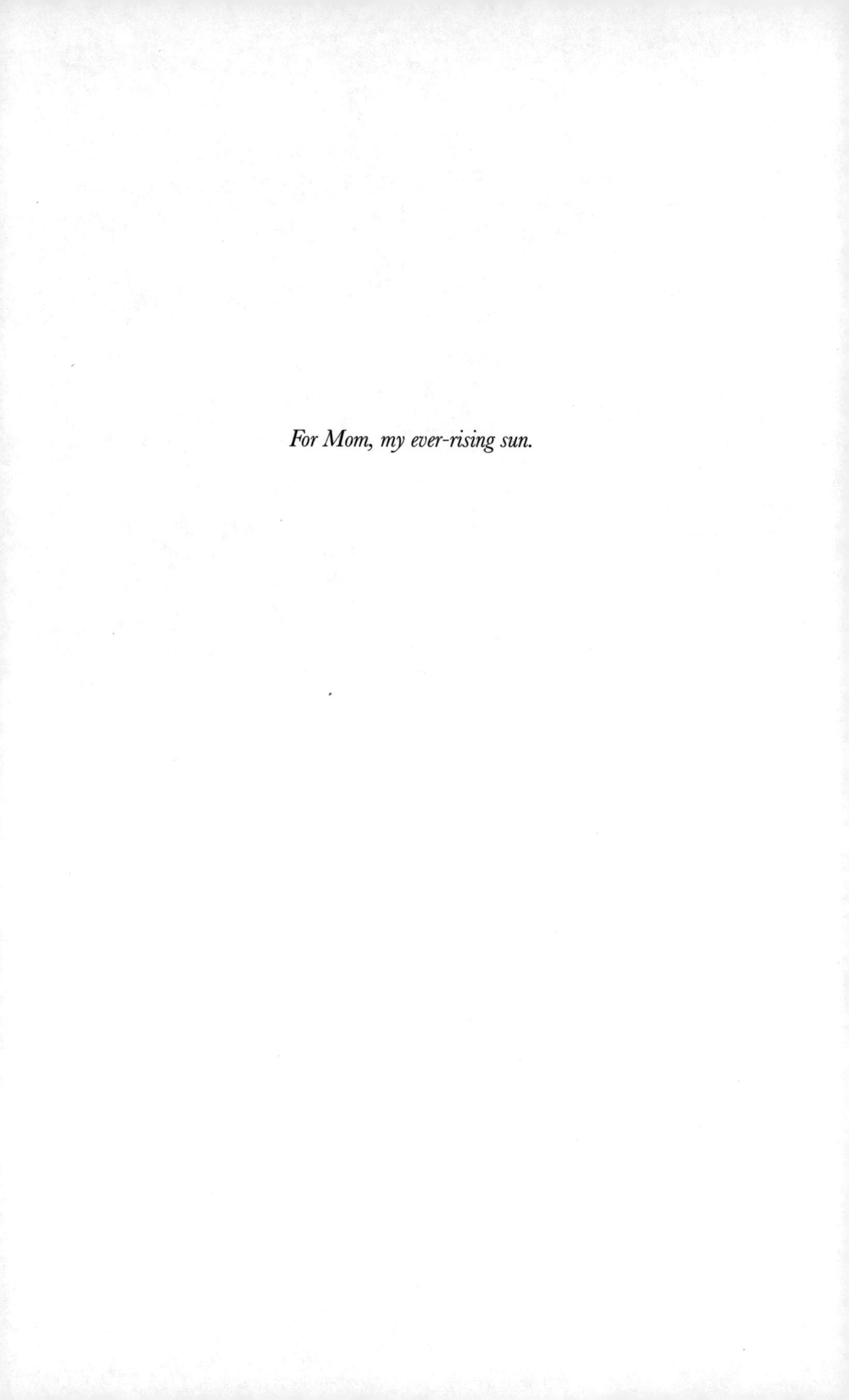

For Mom, my ever-rising sun.

"…from the mystery of night, into the greater mystery of day…"
- Rabindranath Tagore

Reminder

oohwah ooh ooh ooh
oohwah ooh ooh ooh

mourning doves exchange
the same message
across the late morning clearing
and hundreds of years
even the inflections
sometimes
one starts before
the other finishes
still
the same message
the same reply
reminding
balance
territory
you are here with me
the same message
over and over
common knowledge easily forgotten

oohwah ooh ooh ooh
you/are here with me

-Charles Brauer

AUTHOR'S NOTE

In May 2014, I was struck by a car door and flipped over my bicycle handlebars. But the pelvic fracture and months of immobilization were just the beginning of my profound state of undoing. I hadn't just fallen; I'd been pushed. Pushed off the vertiginous edge of all I'd previously known and into deep, uncertain waters.

During recovery, I learned that my deceased, beloved father wasn't my biological father. In the wake of this discovery, just a few months later, my brain rewired itself to perceive solid ground as liquid. This is not a metaphor. My career, like my balance, also went under. Solid footing was a thing of the past. I was out at sea, bobbing, sinking. Weary of chasing cures for my new destabilized reality and running away from my "new" "worse" self, I eventually had to run toward her; I had to return to the beginning—the child's longings, the teenager's compulsions, the young woman's disillusionments—to unwind the history of my identity, and face the concurrent gravity and grace of what it means to live an unfixed, unpolished, unplanned life.

Some call what I experienced a *dark night of the soul*, a *midlife crisis*. Because we have these words for it, I know I'm not alone. The details vary, but most of us have had the feeling—desperately clinging to the last roots of a former identity as the ground crumbles beneath us. Only when life landed me at ground zero, when it dealt me a rare and disruptive condition of perception, was I stripped bare and quiet enough to hear the voice that had been waiting inside me all along.

Our culture is obsessed with fixer uppers—houses, boats, stories. And there are some incredible ones out there. I've spent years and a small fortune wishing mine was one of them. But it wasn't. It isn't. There's been no miracle cure for me. No magic bullet. The magic is elsewhere, though; it's in the commitment to learning how to live well even when the body isn't.

But this process has run counter to a culture that *expects health*, that will go to great lengths—and great expense—to fix what is broken. As a planet, we spend $4.2 trillion annually on health and wellness. This isn't a bad thing. Survival is hardwired into us. But what happens when something breaks that cannot be fixed? When the pills, the treatments, the lifestyle changes all fail? Despite our fix-it culture, many live with chronic illness, pain, and suffering with no cure on the horizon. No easy steps. No life hacks to resolve uncertainty. Beyond the borders of the "fixed" lies a hinterland where pain and disease are not transient but permanent.

And yet, within these shadowy borders, the human spirit often not only prevails—it thrives. It defies logic. When faced with the impossibility of answers, rather than succumb to despair, some find resilience. Some find peace. Some even discover that their brokenness *is* the fix.

At nineteen, I read *The Wisdom of No Escape* by Pema Chödrön. It did not change me—not immediately, at least. I was still a "fix-it" fanatic (and in the decades following, too). But it did plant a seed. It awakened something, or maybe just revealed that another way was possible. But for years, I kept searching for solutions, desperate to make my body, my life, my self *right* again. It took me a long time to realize that the real wisdom wasn't about *fixing* anything—it was about meeting myself exactly where I was. Learning to bear witness to my own suffering, rather than trying to eradicate it, cultivated a patience for the human condition I never had before. As Dr. Rachel Naomi Remen once said, "We thought we could cure everything, but it turns out we can only cure a small amount of disease. The rest of it needs to be held." Every day, I am aware of gravity and my uncertain relationship to it. I have never felt so unstable. And yet, I also feel a growing sense of peace with exactly who I am. A holding of what needs to be held.

For over forty years, this seed has lain dormant within me. Waiting to be nourished, waiting to grow. This memoir is the first rainfall. Sprouts push through, drawn upward by the light of self-reflection, acceptance, and curiosity. What once felt impossible—allowing myself to be as I am, without fixing or forcing—has begun to take root. And like anything which grows toward the sun, I am learning to relax into the reach.

But I've realized growth isn't just forward or upward—it's also downward, inward, backward. Growth is nonlinear; growth is storytelling. As I began to tell my story, I found myself searching for ways to connect with the father I never knew. Though I didn't learn about his identity until after my injury in 2014, I found myself performing a thought experiment: what if my myriad selves— the innocent child, the anxious teenager, the woman still searching—could retroactively relate to him, speak to him somehow? What if I could write this man into being with the knowledge I have *now*, by writing him letters from the perspective of the versions of myself who had no knowledge of him at all? What might have I said to him? How might we have connected? As such, the *Dear Charlie* letters that follow were not written when they're dated, but rather, in the present and as an investigatory way of stepping into the past and allowing it—and me, and him— to breathe. Writing letters from these younger perspectives gave me the freedom to express longings that had never surfaced before, and to weave them into a fuller experience of my current self. The illusory practice of writing directly to him, Charlie, also helped me reflect upon the stories I had learned about him, lean into caring for him, and develop compassion for someone I never had the chance to know.

* * *

The idea of being "unfixed" unsettles some. We resist not having a future self to attain. Some build entire identities around the chase. I was one of them. But for those of us who don't have a choice—and there are so many who don't—there is relief when the chase finally stops. Life emerges right where we are not where we think we should be.

The unfixed see the world differently. Uncertainty becomes a hope. Pain and joy exist simultaneously. They haven't turned their backs on the possibility of answers, but they've learned to live fully despite the lack of one. More often than not, they reorder their lives, prioritizing relationships, creativity, and meaning over status and success. Our biology does everything in its power to fix us. But when it fails, the unfixed adapt. The unfixed tell their stories.

This is mine. Ours.

PART I
HYDROGEN BONDS

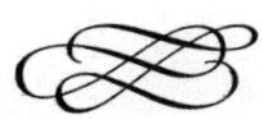

CHAPTER 1

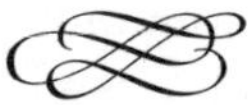

"HE'LL HAVE to drive himself to the airport," Mom says, leaving his flight information on the bathroom counter. The ice in her words cut through the fog of the early morning.

Dad hasn't come home yet. There was a hospital staff party last night—a sendoff for a retiring nurse. He and his surgical partners dressed as famous musicians, singing farewell tunes. Luis Suarez was Julio Iglesias. Trevor Rattray was Harry Belafonte. Dad—already halfway there with his everyday pony tail—was Willie Nelson.

Mom is pissed. Very. She lobs out a few short, pinching remarks —*I'm done forgiving him! He never keeps his commitments!*—then tosses our packed bags into the car. We will fly out without him. Flight 134. Departure time, 6:00 am. He'll have to drive himself to the airport.

We go through security. We board. Then—a neatly folded napkin. A Wisconsin area code scribbled in pen. The flight attendant hands it to Mom with indifference, as if she were handing her a bag of peanuts. I watch her face, searching for any sign. Nothing. I turn to Mom. The furrow in her brow—is that fatigue or worry? Who is trying to contact us at cruising altitude? The long, early-bird drive from our sleepy northern lake town to the Milwaukee airport is always grueling, but the promise of a spring break Mexico sunset in less than twelve hours keeps our spirits lifted. I convince myself that Mom's furrow is indeed fatigue and that everyone receives phone numbers on napkins while flying the friendly skies.

I can't wait to reunite with my brother Eric at the Cancun airport. Every so often, he sends me mixtapes from college—Colorado bands like The Samples and Big Head Todd and the Monsters. To me, his move to Colorado has come with a lifetime membership to cool-dom. Patagonia fleece, Nalgene water bottle in hand—he wears the Rocky Mountain vibe like it was made for him. I try to keep up, slipping into the PowerBar and craft beer tee-shirts he leaves behind, but I swim awkwardly in his castoffs, trying to fit into something too big, too effortlessly cool.

As my butt grows weary on the airplane, cryptic phone number napkin now out of mind, I imagine the big bear hug I'll receive from Eric as he emerges from customs. Dad will match the embrace (and then some) with his famous "four-seconds-too-long" hug.

But the hugs don't come. Instead, when I reunite with Eric, he is falling to his knees. He is crying. The thunder of overstuffed luggage rolling past cannot drown out his sorrow. Not even a little.

I wish I could say I'd felt something, noticed a bird soaring outside our gate's window. Saw a child and father embrace near the Apple Vacations ticketing counter. Something. Anything to mark the moment when, at 5:43am, Dad drove head first into a truck—his soul breaking free from the jaws of life just a half hour behind us on Highway 43, racing to make the flight. Highway 43, right before the two-and road splits into four.

The insignificant little town of Fredonia cradled his crushed ribs that morning as his spirit unfurled its tireless wings. Or maybe they were tired. I don't know.

Highway 43. At 5:43. On April 3. 4/3. He was also born in 1943. This number will follow me. Comfort me. Deceive me. For the rest of my life.

That morning was the first time Mom said "No." No to a twenty-five year dynamic with Dad, one of broken promises and weary forgiveness. No to waiting. No to one more disappointment. That morning we drove to the airport without him.

I want to paint a picture of what I think happened to Dad that foggy April morning. I want to trace his thoughts. Did he feel abandoned by us when he returned home from the party? Did he feel guilty? Was he sleepy from a previous day of life-saving or was he drunk from a night of Willie and wine? Was he happy? When he pulled into the garage, he would have already known that Mom and I had left. I know he was in a hurry because we saw, twenty hours later, his clothes tossed on the bed in a frenzy to pack for a week in Mexico. I bet he packed in less than five minutes, remembering all the necessities—wallet, pager, and that bristle brush he loved for a good head scratching. I know he saw Mom's note—*MEET US IN MEXICO. I'M PISSED.* Underline. Underline. Underline. I know this because the county police found it in the passenger seat of his totaled car. They briefly investigated a possible homicide.

So, in less than five minutes, he grabbed the note, traded briefcase for luggage, maybe chugged a glass of water in the kitchen. That's it. So why, then—why—did he take time to scotch tape a cartoon from yesterday's *New York Times* onto the bathroom mirror? We found it on the bottom left corner, just above his bar of sandalwood soap. A line drawing of a bearded man, weary, scaling the face of a steep mountain. The caption beneath him read: *Life is but a game. Too bad the batteries aren't included.*

I stand at Mom's side after we pass through customs, watching as she dials the number on the napkin. It doesn't take long for the operator to connect her—unknowingly—to her widowed destiny. Mom glances at me sideways; I know this look. She's irritated because I'm not near our luggage. Let the Texans have my flip-flops, my new spring-break sundress. I need to be *here*, anchored beside her as she makes first contact with the human on the other end of the line. Not to comfort her, but to steal a moment of control. Something isn't right. I claim the floor beneath my feet, claiming its solidity. I don't budge. Then— the floor is quick sand. My head spins. Am I about to pass out? My brain pounds with vacant incomprehension as Mom's lipstick-stained mouth forms the words, "Dad's dead."

The only thing keeping me from blacking out is a thin membrane of awareness. The persistent roar of luggage. The hum of voices moving this way, then that. A woman laughing.

Instead of my body going limp and surrendering to the plump, grandmotherly arms of a passing tourist, I freeze. I don't know it at the time, but this is what trauma therapists mean by *fight, flight or freeze.* I am clearly of the popsicle variety.

Cold deadens to numbness. Numbness erases sensation, removes it from my reach. And somewhere in this slow, slipping away, denial builds a home inside me. For the next twelve hours I convince myself that Mom is *nuts*, Eric is *dramatic*, and Dad is safe at home smoking a pipe and reading Ann Rice. I dissociate. My breath comes in small, shallow gasps—if I inhale too deeply, everything will collapse.

On the flight back to the Midwest, I sit beside Eric, my headphones cocooning me inside his latest mix. Some weed-induced moment back at CU Boulder probably inspired his hand written title, but I'm struck now by its new and eerie poignancy: *Time Stood Still.* I listen to Bob Marley's *High Tide or Low* on repeat, drowning out the panic pressing against my ribs. Later, I'll listen to the song—forever the soundtrack to The Day Dad Died—and try to decode it, searching for a message from beyond, an attempt to make meaning from the ambivalence of life.

We land in Chicago. Fat snowflakes swirl through the air, muffling the world, quieting the scream in my gut. We have a four-hour drive ahead. Mom slows as we pass through Fredonia, its streets buried under fresh drifts. A kind flight attendant had slipped her some sleeping pills on our flight back. I took half of one, and now I feel the drug push into me like a heavy snowfall.

Distant farmhouses glow as winter asserts her strength over spring. Just another day here. That morning, tired wives bought pastries at the local bakery, children hid in haylofts until the school bus arrived. By evening, the town has sealed itself away in warmth.

We pull over where Dad's car skidded into oblivion less than 24 hours ago. The snow has already erased his tracks.

I step out of the car. The ground is slick, and for a brief moment, I feel it—one wrong move and I could slip through too. When someone dies, does a thin veil lift between dimensions? A quiet invitation? How long does it stay open?

Mom suggests we hold hands and scream. We scream so loud I swear I see lights flicker on in neighboring houses. And for the first time in my adolescent, self-conscious world, *I don't care.* I am desperate for something real. A lone wolf calling to her pack.

Snowflakes fall on my face as I tilt my head back, listening for Dad's response.

Nothing.

I crawl into the back seat of the car and shrink into silent fantasy. I visualize the garage door opening at home, Dad's license plate "YANG" mocking us as we pull aside it. The more I burn this vision into my brain, the louder Mom and Eric's cries become. I want out of the car. I hate them for being loud and emotional. *There is no room for me.* I don't know how I need to respond but I don't want to do it their way. I become smaller and smaller in the back seat and eventually slip out from under my seatbelt, out the crack in the window, and into the arms of Dad.

After pulling into the empty garage, I collapse, my journal clutched to my chest. I stare at my hands, willing them to become his.

Magical thinking consumes me.

I make a pact: his hands will work through mine.

I will take his path where his abbreviated life could not.

APRIL 3, 1993

Dear Charlie,

This morning, 4/3 at 5:43, on Highway 43, Dad's car collided with a Mac truck. He's dead. I feel numb. I feel nothing. Earlier today Mom, Eric and I were at the Cancun airport. She led us outside to a pink, flowering bush and knelt down in the dusty earth. She asked us to join her. I was numb. I felt nothing. If she had asked me to swallow an iguana whole, I would've said yes. Just tell me what to do.

While happy flowers ridiculed our reality, Mom said that Dad wants us to live our lives fully. I don't know what this means.

I'm in the meditation room now. We have one in our house. Pretty cool. But pretty sad, now, too. It smells like Dad. We've traveled over 6000 miles in less than 24 hours. When we left home, I was thinking about blue Gulf of Mexico waters and the new pimple on my chin. Now, here I am. Numb. I can't remember anything from today except Dad's request—or was it Mom's?

Dad wants us to live our lives fully.

There was an anesthesiologist from Appleton Medical Center driving behind him. He recognized Dad's car and vanity plate. He said moments before the collision, Dad reached his hand through the sun roof and waved to the rising sun. Was he waving hello? Or was he waving goodbye?

Does his spirit exit stubbornly, clinging to ribcage and bone, or was he squeezed out like toothpaste from a phantom umbilicus? Maybe some rise easily, like the yeasty force of leavened bread, warmed to meet a new infinite celling. Maybe others catch on spinning fans and ride out eternity on a dizzy blade.

Or is it simpler than all of this? After car crushes, heart ceases, breath escapes, I mistake his now vacant body—its yawning void—for a soul. I name it, I animate it, I call for it—but it's only so my own void has a place to go.

CHAPTER 2

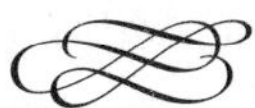

SATURDAY AFTERNOON, summer of 1974, Mom and her friend Lynn are watching a glass blowing demonstration, lounging in the grass, and listening to a local folk singer's lilting ballads. Later, they will meander the festival grounds in search of a snack. The solstice celebration at the Mariposa Folk Festival on the Toronto Islands hums with the easy, golden rhythm of long daylight and warm music. The two had been itching for an adventure, away from the cold of southern Michigan. Here at the festival, Ann Arbor feels a world away.

Near the food vendors, a young musician leans against a tree, strumming his guitar like it's an old friend. As Mom and Lynn pass within earshot, he lifts his head and starts to sing:

"You're much too pretty, for me to just a'walk up and say hi…»

Mom catches his gaze, startled, amused.

"But if I don't you'd probably just a'walk on by…"

She nudges Lynn, suppressing a grin. The man doesn't break eye contact, strumming gently, his voice kind and teasing.

"I've been seeing ya for a long, long while. I don't know your name, oh but I know your smile…"

Mom laughs now, caught up in the game. She flashes him her own wide, toothy song.

"And I'd really liiiiiiiiiike to get to know you."

The last note hangs in the warm air as he strums a final chord, then steps forward, extending a hand.

"Hi. Name's Charles. You can call me Charlie." His voice has a playful, faintly southern drawl, easy as the summer afternoon.

Mom, usually soured by flirtatious men, finds herself leaning in instead. There's something boyish about him, something open and unaffected. She shakes his hand without reservation.

"I'm Nancy," Mom offers, then gestures toward her friend as an afterthought. "This is Lynn." Charlie whistles to someone nearby, waving him over. With a knowing nudge, he steers the newcomer toward Lynn.

"Beer?," he asks Mom. Before she can answer, he perches his guitar up against the tree and starts collecting abandoned cups, pouring their remains into one cup until it's full. He hands her the communal beer. She hesitates, then accepts—charmed more by his carefree swagger than his back-wash brew. They settle onto the grass, taking small sips. Charlie talks—his words relaxed, animated—about music, history, the natural world. He tells her about the show he hosts on Wisconsin Public Television, *Long Ago is All Around,* where he and his dog, Ranger, teach kids about the state's past.

Charlie also mentions his recent graduation from U of M Ann Arbor—an odd coincidence—and Mom is jolted from the otherwise carefree exchange. Her mind is briefly elsewhere: a tall, handsome cardiac resident walking the Ann Arbor campus at this very moment. He is shadowing doctors; he is flirting with nurses. *As this stranger charms me*, she thinks, *is my husband back on campus charming someone else*?

During her first pregnancy some years ago, David Warner—my dad—started having affairs. Mom knew about them. And for now, they'd ended. But when she attends the 1974 Mariposa Festival, she thinks she might be pregnant again and has an appointment with her OBGYN when she returns; during the long drive between Ann Arbor and Toronto, she wonders if the affairs will start all over again with the news of their second child.

But she is tired of being "Parson Larson." As a child her most intimate, late night conversations were with a portrait of Christ hanging on her bedroom wall. As a young woman she held Bible studies in her college dorm room. Her first kiss with Dad was unintentionally shared with a Bible—positioning their torsos a safe three inches apart—as they embraced on a shady path of their Wooster College campus.

Now, a young wife and mother, she struggles to apply Christ's teachings of forgiveness in her marriage. Throw in a classic 1950's attitude about keeping up appearances and fear of being alone and she is in it for the long haul. But on this early summer day, something breaks in her. Maybe it's the communal beer and the spirit of the 70s. Maybe it's the sudden urge to color outside the lines and know herself without borders.

So that night, sandwiched between star and beer cup constellations, I am conceived.

* * *

Mom and Dad sit at the dinner table. She doesn't waste time.

"Dave, I need to tell you…I had sex with a man last night."

Dad shoves peas around his plate. Doesn't look up. His thoughts seem to be sorted into a logical, legume-shaped blockade, separating emotion from reason. Finally, he lifts his gaze. Sheepish. Hurt.

"I, I don't know what to say."

The silence stretches. Long enough for the wall clock's second hand to regulate both their heartbeats.

"Nance, I know don't have the right to be angry."

He doesn't ask for details. Doesn't touch the words she's placed between them. They continue eating, burying what's been said.

We shape our narratives from the known details of our lives. But hidden truths—the ones we bury—shape us too. Sometimes more powerfully than we care to admit. Truth is a persistent, nocturnal companion who needs daylight to survive. In this story, my story, the companion's name is Charlie.

A week later, Mom stacks cans of tuna in the pantry of their Ann Arbor rental. My three-year old brother Eric throws pick-up sticks across the kitchen floor between her shopping bags. As she bends to gather them, a confident *tap, tap, tap* sounds at the front screen door. Mom is an extrovert and has already settled into a circle of friends in their new life in Michigan. Assuming it's one of these new friends dropping by for a chat, she walks to the door—then stops short. On the other side of the screen stands a familiar, sunny-faced young man.

"Hi Nancy!" Charlie's voice is earnest, lyrical. The weekend at the Mariposa Festival floods her, eddies of caution and thrill spiral into her core.

"Charlie! What a surprise!" she says, masking her trepidation with a cheery welcome and swings the door open. A thousand unspoken questions flicker through her mind. *How did he find me? Did I give him this address in a moment of careless abandon? Did I even tell him my last name? Do I know his?*

They sit at the kitchen table and make small talk in the face of big feelings. Eric bounces easily on Mom's lap, then Charlie's. In the pedestrian light of a weekday kitchen, they are strangers to each other—friendly strangers. Charlie is easy with himself and his surroundings, putting Mom at ease as well.

"My husband, Dave, knows about us. I told him the night I came home."

Charlie nods steadily, revealing nothing. *Does his heart sink in this moment or is it unleashed—a wild dog catching the scent of something just out of reach?*

"There is no room for more exploration." She continues, words careful but firm. "And what I really need to do is work on my marriage."

A slow-burning shame creeps into her cheeks as she takes him in—this openhearted, spirited young man, so *young*. A recent college graduate. She, on the other hand, is an almost thirty-year-old woman with a toddler and marital problems. She doesn't want to hurt him. He seems confident, easy, but is he?

Charlie holds her gaze. Then, with a grin that lands somewhere between playful and unreadable, he shrugs. "That's alright. But it's a gorgeous day—how about a picnic? I hitchhiked all the way over here. Got nothing else to do."

Mom's hands are full with a restless toddler—how could she possibly go on a picnic? But it *is* a beautiful summer day, and

Charlie says he has access to a private pond with a cabin and canoe. She thinks, *I can do this. It's innocent. Friendly.* So they pack some towels, a change of diapers and clothes for Eric, and pile into Mom's car. They stop at a corner market, pick up cheese, salami, a baguette.

Nothing remarkable happens that day, unless you are more of the poetic mind and believe that sunshine, a canoe and three humans enjoying each other's company *is* remarkable.

Later in life, Eric will joke, "I checked out your dad that day. He was a good guy."

Charlie's lightheartedness is a welcome contrast to Dad's serious, studious nature. There are no expectations here. No secrets. But hidden just below the surface of this unassuming, sun-drenched scene, there aren't three humans in the canoe, but *four*—one embryonic, unknown—cradled in the warmth of a perfect Midwestern summer day.

Reaching up to rest a hand on my chest now, I listen to the solid thump of my heart and wonder—on that day, did the tiny fertilized egg nestled into Mom's uterine wall undergo a rapid and ecstatic cellular division as she recognized the laughter of her origins?

* * *

A few years later, I am five, tucked into the corner of the family room sofa, a cheese sandwich gripped in my greasy hands, watching Wisconsin Public Television. I am fixated on a blond, charismatic man singing songs about the history of our state, his dog Ranger at his feet. Mom walks in and sees Charlie and me staring at each other through a phosphorescent screen and stops in her tracks. The three of us hold a brief, televised communion.

SEPTEMBER 23, 1985

Dear Charlie,

I came home from school today, ate a bowl of Cheerios and swam in the lake. Lake Winnebago, that is. I know it's late in the summer to be swimming—or is it already fall? It certainly feels like it today. But I can't resist being tossed by chilly whitecaps, the near-nakedness of my body swallowed and reborn by my wet, temperamental friend.

You set out over stormy waters today too. I hope that when you left the shores of Frankfurt, Michigan, your belly was warm from both feast and friends. I hope that the waters of Lake Michigan, only a few hundred miles from my inland puddle, embraced you with the 360 degrees of aliveness you were seeking, your sails loyal to the distant shore, but your heart caught happily somewhere in between.

I wonder if we were reborn at the same time.

CHAPTER 3

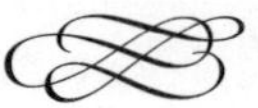

LAKE WINNEBAGO IS NOT JUST a body of water. It's a family member. Algonquian tribes called their Ho Chunk neighbors inhabiting the shores of this shallow, freshwater lake near the eastern border of Wisconsin the Winnebagos. This translates to "people of the filthy water." I love the filth—the thick, green sludge that accumulates in summertime waters.

August swimming lines my suit with fertile, photosynthetic organisms. I peel my one-piece off and wash the green from my skin, but I'm not repulsed like my friends. These waters are my amniotic fluid, my sustenance. I swim when I'm happy. I swim when I'm sad. When weather stirs the water into whitecaps, I throw my body into their walls of unapologetic power. When the surface is glass, I sit cross-legged on the sandy bottom and listen to a murky underworld.

Only later in life will we question the magnitudes of algae —the inevitable explosion of life from agricultural run-off. Fertilizers and pesticides have steadily polluted these waters, suffocating the natural balance of aquatic life. But innocence is bliss. To me, the warm stench and the bobbing balls of neon blue-green are an integral part of childhood. They *are* childhood. My senses are at once assaulted by and surrendered to Lake Winnebago's reckless cycles of life and death.

I wonder why it's so easy for me to surrender in water. In my terrestrial existence, I am willful and persistent. "By self!"—one of the first sentences to throw itself from my young vocal cords—was used with authority for years. I love having a goal, turning off all other distractions and forging toward it. I wave my magic wand and make the impossible possible.

One windy winter day, Mom and Dad step into their cross-country skis, setting off across the fresh powder along the frozen shore of Winnebago. Mom loops a rope around her waist, threading it through the front of a plastic sled, and I plop my five-year old body into my purple chariot. She glides forward, her legs cutting smooth tracks in the snow, and I sink into the rhythm, letting the landscape press its slow, barren story into my vision. The wind chill bites below zero, winter exhaling onto the pink circumference of my exposed cheeks. Dad's mustache is filled with snot-cicles. Mom's tiny waist and ample hips sway back and forth in her red, one-piece jumper.

From a distance, I spot a brown, skipping shape across the horizon. An early Easter bunny? A large squirrel? It moves erratically, wind-tossed yet determined, bounding in our direction. Mom angles toward the shoreline, reaching just as it tangles in the low, bony branches of a tree. She is a ruby promise amidst a vast landscape of white, harsh sleep. Bending down, she untangles the object—now crumpled, small in her fist, and shoves it into her pocket. But as she turns to look back at me, it snags on her ski pole strap and is free again. This time, a strong, westward gust seizes it, hurling it back in my direction.

I watch it blow past me, not a bunny or a squirrel, but a baggie from the local Piggly Wiggly market. Mom calls out "Grab it Kimmy!" but inside my snow suit, my limbs move—or don't— like they are encased in marshmallow fluff. My eyes, uninhibited, track the bag, priming my limbic system to do what it loves to do. One moon-boot in front of the other, I roll out of the sled and start plodding through snow as high as my waist, never losing sight of my prey.

Mom calls out through the blasting, sideways gusts, "Leave it be! Come back!" But I can't. Time, will, and the limitations of flesh will determine the baggie's fate now.

I chant out loud, "I think I can. I think I can." Eyes fixed. Legs lifting in and out of thick powder. The snow makes my legs impossibly heavy. The wind shoves me in the other direction. I start to feel cold from the inside out and a dull ache rises from my belly that longs to be near Mom again. But I don't give up; the pull of pursuit grips me tight. Just feet below my boots, the ice shifts as a crack begins to form between my will and my want. My mind says go forward, my flesh says go back. *I think I can, I think I can.*

But the hot, damp breath inside my scarf is hypnotic comfort. The slow, rhythmic crunch of my boots is my beat. As long as I have my eyes on the goal, I feel connected to everything, playing my part in Winnebago's Waltz of the Snow Flakes.

The baggie eventually finds another tree to tangle into, and its fate is mine. I continue chanting "I think I can, I think I can," watching it flap helplessly against a broken branch. Once it's within arm's reach, I stop—the first pause since the chase began. My face is numb, but I want to savor this moment. When it slipped from Mom's pocket, it was full of possibility—east, west, north and south, all unwritten chapters. Now its destiny is in my hand. But I don't want it yet. The reward isn't Mom's appreciation. It isn't the flimsy plastic bag. If my legs weren't tired, my cheeks raw from the wind, I'd knock it loose and keep going, high on my own pharmacological edition of *The Little Engine That Could*. The reward is the chase. And now that it's over, I feel empty.

SEPTEMBER 24, 1985

Dear Charlie,

I was late again for the school bus so Mom in her bathrobe, with a slippered foot heavy on the gas pedal, chased it halfway to Electa Quinney Elementary. I know the driver saw Mom maniacally flashing her headlights while kids in the back of the bus laughed and pointed accusatory fingers. But she was determined to punish my mom, her mom, and all moms for ever being late. My stomach tied itself in knots when she finally stopped long enough for the awkward dash between the warmth of the car and the bus aisle's walk of shame. While looking for an empty seat, the red in my cheeks deepening, I pictured my refuge at the bottom of the lake. Cold, silent, peaceful.

I didn't know you were already there.

CHAPTER 4

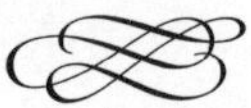

The Open Marriage, by Nena and George O'Neill, was a bestseller in the 1970s. The book aimed to "strip marriage of its antiquated ideals and romantic tinsel" proposing that non-monogamous exploration could foster personal growth and ultimately save a struggling marriage.

I am three-and-a-half-years-old when a therapist introduces this book to Mom and Dad—an antidote or last ditch effort, I'm not sure—to help them navigate their murky infidelities. After careful consideration, they decide it's their best chance at saving the family. The open marriage lasts for five years.

Even as a child, I sense that our family isn't like others. Most parents don't rewrite the rules of marriage. This is not happening in my best friend Jenny's churchgoing household.

I remember Mom and Dad as happy; until happiness combusts. Loving, until love turns volatile. They are respectful and affectionate in public. When they reunite at the end of a work day, all 6'6" of Dad's charismatic frame rises to greet Mom with a kiss. At the dinner table, their conversation is engaged until Mom dumps her salad bowl on Dad's head and Dad throws his water at her face.

They work long hours but also make time to relax, travel, attend workshops at Esalen—a retreat center in Big Sur, California known for personal growth and live-work residencies. There, they study with wellness pioneers like Brugh Joy and Rachel Naomi Remen, immersing themselves in mind-body medicine and transpersonal psychology. Our library at home overflows with books on healing, consciousness, and the limitless potential of the human spirit.

Family vacations are frequent, as are the verbal boxing matches that break out when we spend too much time together. Long car rides are torture. The invisible line I draw between us does nothing, protects nothing, so I defend myself by *becoming* nothing—an undetectable survival strategy misinterpreted at Sweet, Pleasing Kimmy.

When loud and angry voices ricochet off the wood floors and walls, I hide in my bedroom, shrinking down into tiny, imperceptible breaths. As their voices rise, mine diminishes. They take up space as I get small. This shrink-wrapped version of myself is good at muffling the cavernous fear in my gut. I strain to hear one of them say "divorce" or "it's over" bracing for the inevitable, but the storms pass and then—just like that—they seem happy again. The cycle is circuitous and unsustainable. But at the time, I just see it as them trying. I see it as them loving one another.

Mom and Dad attend "relationship workshops" around the world more frequently than most parents visit the car wash. And when they return, psyches scrubbed clean, there is more kissing in the kitchen and Wednesday afternoons behind a locked bedroom door—sometimes even new wedding bands. Mom's jewelry box smells like salty metal and amber; I like opening it up, filling my nose with familiarity and then dragging my fingers, *clink clink clink*, through the shiny, musical shapes. My favorite ring is a simple gold band that has "Y APE OU" engraved on the inside. I have no idea what it means but I like saying it over and over in my head. Sometimes the vowels are long and soothing. Sometimes they sound like a war cry.

This is Mom and Dad's first wedding band from their early twenties. I don't want to ask Jenny if her parents have multiple rings. I'm embarrassed by my family. We don't fit the mold. But I do like my parents' multiple ring tradition. Especially because, each time they get a new one, they seem happy again.

One night, while Mom tucks me in, I ask her what "Y APE

OU" means. She smiles. "It was our way of saying 'I love you.' But 'love'—real love—is more than romance. It's *agape, philos,* and *eros* all together—divine love, friendship, and desire." She pauses, then laughs, smoothing my blanket. "We wanted something bigger than a fairytale. Bigger than what the church expected from a good Christian couple." Then pauses with a knowing grin, "Be careful what you ask for."

In their last year of the open marriage, Dad quits his heart surgery practice and moves for a while to Esalen. I hear other kids in school talk about divorce and wonder again if this is where my family is headed. Dad exits my world smelling of antiseptic hospital soap; six months later, he returns in an aura of ylang ylang and tobacco.

Mom drives to Appleton's small municipal airport to pick him up, but pulling into Arrivals she is looking for the wrong man. Dad swaggers into the passenger seat wearing a black leather jacket, his hair pulled into a long pony-tail and a cigarette hangs casually from his mouth. She passes a Motel 6 and wonders if it would be a better drop-off point for this strange man than bringing him home to begin yet another new chapter of marriage.

Dad returns to Appleton Medical Center (AMC) but after his long hiatus, he's forbidden from performing surgery. Instead, he's back to interning on a 32K salary, trailing his former partners around the hospital like a dropout medical student. I imagine he's embarrassed—but maybe a little thrilled? He always loved breaking the rules.

At Esalen, he studied meditation, breathwork and mind-body medicine, and now he brings home some new tricks. Research is starting to draw connections between cardiac health and stress management, and Dad is at the forefront of introducing this movement to AMC. But to a conservative Midwestern hospital, his "radical" ideas aren't just unwelcome—they're threatening. He comes home from work increasingly defeated.

Sometimes I play with his biofeedback machine, strapping my index finger into a device that measures peripheral blood circulation. I breathe deeply, imagining myself submerged in warm water and try to turn the light from blue to red. But either the machine is faulty or I am. It's always blue.

During the open marriage, Mom and Dad were encouraged to communicate openly about their sexual encounters—nurturing intimacy by sharing their intimacies. Mom, with her insatiable curiosity and near Vulcan-like ability to transmute discomfort into inquiry, leads most of these conversations. She learns about Dad's string of one-night-stands with nurses at the hospital, flirtations with friends and strangers. He, on the other hand, wants no details about Mom's affairs.

Not until years after the open marriage ends does Dad learn that Mom had only one relationship in those five, long years—a man she grew to love. But instead of abandoning ship, Mom and Dad hoist their sails and go back to sea. They have new wedding bands made. Will these be the last?

They also start teaching relationship workshops, determined to unearth meaning and purpose from their painful story. Dad draws from his western medical knowledge and newfound passion for natural medicine; Mom brings her marriage and family counseling skills to the table. On Sundays they haul sharpies and large, colorful blotting boards into the meditation room (formerly Dad's office, now outfitted with an altar, crystals and Angel Cards—the perfect New Age facelift) and condense years of pain, angst, curiosity and courage into hope.

But when I ask Mom if she'd ever recommend an open marriage to struggling couples, she doesn't hesitate.

"No way."

AUGUST 15, 1986

Dear Charlie,

I'm on Rock Island this week with Mom, her friends, their kids, and of course, Jenny. We fell asleep last night to the lulling white noise of rain on the tent, but my dreams are restless.

In one, I wandered alone to Rock Island's old stone boat dock—the one Jenny and I are convinced is haunted. The moon was high, its light fractured by moving clouds, but everything around me was steeped in shadow. I sat on the dock's edge, my feet dangling over water, watching their reflection in the black glass below. No sound, not even the gentle lap of waves against stone, as if someone had turned the volume off in my dream.

I stayed that way for a long time staring at the oily, black reflection of my feet. Everything was dark; even the dock's grey stones were deep charcoal. The lake stretched endlessly, a void, swallowing all light. Almost. As if a novice painter had misplaced the light source, my nightgown remained bright as daylight—a celestial body adrift in a sea of black.

And then I saw another light, far below my feet. A peaceful shape, resting, with Lake Michigan as its eternal blanket. I lowered myself onto my belly, hanging my head over the dock to see more clearly. My nightgown's glow stretched toward the water searching for its other half. I felt magnetically pulled, as if something below was calling to me.

As I inched closer, the shapes took form. Bones. A man. Long femurs, wide ribs, curled up into the quiet, protective shape of a fetus. Born a circle, we live ourselves into lines and then relinquish them back into a circle.

His arms rested peacefully over his ribs, but I knew, without question, that they were also reaching—stretching upward, back to me.

CHAPTER 5

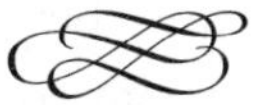

EVERY YEAR, Mom and a few of her mom-friends organize a camping trip to Rock Island. What began as a feminist "Who needs testosterone?" challenge has become an anticipated and cherished tradition. Each mom plans a breakfast, lunch and dinner, or enough for a few days depending on how long we stay. This isn't the pared-down Outward Bound backpacking I will learn about in my late teens. There are no cars on Rock Island, but we aren't exactly roughing it. We drive caravan-style to the tip of Door County, take a car ferry to Washington Island, then leave our cars behind and board a passenger-only ferry that finally lands us on Rock Island. Coolers brimming with food make the journey with us. And we have access to fresh water from the island's boathouse pump and share outhouses with horse flies.

Days unfold in a flurry of eager limbs, beach towels, and the bottomless hunger of children set loose in summer. Nights are spent by the fire, skin pruned from hours in the lake, laughter rising between bites of burnt marshmallow, the air thick with smoke, stories, and song.

I love Lake Michigan the way I love Lake Winnebago—not as intimately, but with a deep and abiding familiarity. I only spend a week each summer in its cool, deep waters, yet those yawning

Mediterranean-blue lake days have embedded themselves in my DNA. Lake Michigan's water feels different on my skin than Lake Winnebago's. It's silky, invigorating. I dive under and open my eyes, seeing at least ten feet below my toes. It's cold but as soon as my head is wet, I acclimatize and float for hours, held by water so giant and deep that it takes me a few moments to overcome my fear—but only a few moments. Once I am reacquainted with this distant relative, we are inseparable. I pull her mysterious waters into my dreams. I weigh down my sweatshirt pockets with her large, smooth stones. I sneak little sips of her impossibly clear body, pretending I'm drinking some exotic elixir of immortality.

CHAPTER 6

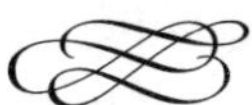

WHILE SCANNING Mom and Dad's ever-growing self-help library, I grab a book titled *Dying to Live* by Tolly Burkan, founder of the international fire-walking movement. I'm twelve. Earlier that June, our family attended his workshop in Canada, and on the final evening, participants were invited to walk barefoot across burning embers. It sounded like magic to me.

I'd heard of walking on water but that was reserved for the guy I occasionally read about in Sunday school with Jenny, flipping through the Bible just enough to appear *normal* to her family. But fire walking? That was something else entirely.

Tolly's bright blue eyes, ablaze with his own internal fire, evangelized his message for ordinary people like me—if you can walk on fire, you can do anything. Through sharing his own story of suffering and transformation, he made happiness and freedom sound almost… easy. His recipe simple: *Pay attention. Expect the best. Go for it.*

I was too young, and they had rules about youth "going for it," so I watched Mom, Dad and Eric join the others, ungracefully scooting across hot coals.

I didn't inspect everyone's feet the next morning, but charred flesh wouldn't dissuade me. I was obsessed. Tolly was my first introduction to the "human potential" movement and those two, insignificant words shoved together in my brain were like a match to dry tinder.

In his book, I learn that fire-walking is an exercise in relaxing the body and mind so that the perception of pain is *simply* an intense sensation—neither good nor bad. He claims that if the brains react *Yikes, we're in danger,* you're more likely to get burned, and those who stay relaxed make it across unscathed.

So, my thoughts and state of mind can determine my physical reality? I'm thrilled—the vaccine to an unpredictable, painful world right inside my own head. I sift through my memory, scanning for moments of pain. Stomach aches—bad. Dog bites, corrective orthodontics bites, Eric's perfected Spock bites (also known as the Vulcan Nerve Pinch)—bad, bad, bad. Can I really have ultimate control over it all? It seems only natural to judge an intense sensation or experience as bad and figure out how to avoid it. But Tolly is telling me something different. He is saying I can take away pain's power. He's saying *I'm in control.*

I close the book triumphantly and make a plan. *If I'm too young to firewalk, then I'll do the next best thing.*

Most summer days are spent splashing in Lake Winnebago with Jenny, building miniature kingdoms from cardboard and found objects (with Jenny), and playing with dolls and ignoring impending puberty (with Jenny). Everything I do is with Jenny. We have been inseparable since our first secret, shoe-lace tying race in first grade. So I'm not certain why I am alone on this early summer day when I march outside with a mission.

I decide I need to walk barefoot around the perimeter of the house, testing my coltish feet against the petrified wood stumps that line the path down to the lake. I'm used to being barefoot in the summer, proud of the thick tomboy callouses that come with it. This isn't just a game—it's an experiment, a way to prove that I'm in control of my body.

Pay attention. Expect the best. Go for it.

I hurl my right foot forward, slamming it against the edge of the rock-hard stump, convinced that I can experience stubbing my toe as a pure sensation—neither good nor bad. Expecting the best means I will transcend pain, free from suffering at last.

I do it again with my left foot. Then my right again. Again. And again. My inner drill sergeant is relentless. I am stubborn. Willful. Determined to win this invisible war.

I think I can, I think I can.

Thirty minutes later, my toes are bleeding. I wanted to know if I could rewire my brain's response—that the sharp, insistent throb in my nerves wasn't a warning, just a sensation. I wanted to feel the hot pulse inside my toes as a rhythm, a dance party in my feet. I wanted to prove that pain— inevitable, unpredictable—was under my control.

But I couldn't do it. *I think I can; I know I can't.*

Conclusion of my grand experiment? Being in a body hurts.

Not long after my experiment I notice a deep, bruised sensation just below my knee caps. My heart is also bruised. After six inseparable years, Jenny's family moves to Tennessee. I deny it until the last possible moment—until the moving van pulls away.

That morning, I bike the 2.5 miles between our homes through a late-summer drizzle, convinced that when I arrive, nothing will have changed. We'll skip into the kitchen, steal two Hostess Ho Ho's —unrolling them to eat the cream first—then wiggle our eager minds and bodies into endless play. Instead, I arrive to an empty house. Jenny stands at the door, her eyes bloodshot and tired. We hug, I'm sure we hug, but I don't remember anything else until the large moving truck disappears, the family car trailing behind, Jenny's face craning to look out the back window.

I bike home and bury my head in Mom's lap, sobbing so hard I swear my skull will crack under pressure. The ache comes from my toes, travels through my guts and out my eyes. Pain is no longer a subject under the lens of my microscope. Pain suddenly is very real. I hear its jagged edges escape from my throat and I float outside myself to a safer place.

Years later, I will remember this moment as if watching it from above. There's a girl curled in fetal position on her mom's lap. There's her sadness, so deep it is indistinguishable from the love she feels for her friend. By letting the sorrow flood through her, there she is, writing her best friend's name—JENNY— in permanent ink on her heart, never to fade.

The bruising on my knees deepens, then swells. Large, unsightly bumps develop just below my kneecaps, tender to the slightest shift in gravity—each step a hammer strike, each movement a dull, relentless jab. *Osgood Schlatters* is what the doctor calls it but there's nothing "Os-good" about it. I'm told it's common in active adolescents—the constant tug of muscle on tendon irritating the growth plate beneath the knee. At the time of diagnosis, I am a leaping, jumping, running, swimming, hand-standing, pirouetting ribbon of flesh. And now, I'm told, all of it must to come to a screeching halt until the rapid growth spurt subsides.

I spend my time remediating on the hard bench at the front of the ballet studio—me and a handful of distracted stage moms. My envy swells in proportion to the height of my classmates' graceful extensions. I convince myself that when I return to the barre, I too will have grown stronger, more fluid, as if grace can be willed into existence through longing alone. I ache for the deceptive ease that flows from a dancer's body, knowing full well the battle of muscle and ligament waging just beneath the surface is part of what makes it so compelling.

Six months later, the pain begins to diminish. Pliés are fine but grande pliés still feel like someone has stuffed smooth rocks below my knee caps. Maybe Jenny put them there because I can't separate the pain in my knees from the pain of missing her. But the pursuit of muscular precision to the soundtrack of Chopin and Tchaikovsky eventually buries those rocks. I become obsessed with the world of ballet. Nothing is ever good enough and this gives me a reason to keep pushing. *The reward is the chase.* Dad is my resident sports masseuse, working the unnatural poses out of my muscles with his strong hands and the occasional found tool when his fingers grow weary—a kitchen fork, a rock from the lake, a racquetball—talismans of every day that bury my pain so deeply I eventually forget it exists.

But I'm not made for ballet. At least physically. I outgrow

everyone in my class—my long arms, legs and feet never gain the control that Balanchine dancer Gelsey Kirkland flawlessly executes in my favorite documentary *Dancing with Mr. B.* My ribcage is too big, my shoulders too wide. My Russian ballet trained instructor, Jaunita Makaroff (who we revere and fear in equal measure) makes no adjustments for physical attributes that reject her standards. "Ribs in Kim! Shoulders down!" But what I don't have structurally I make up for mentally. I crave the discipline that ballet provides. It channels all my tendencies for obsessive compulsiveness.

Throughout childhood and adolescence I trade one, repetitive behavior for another—my inner chaos leaking to the surface. Squeezing my shoulders up and down, stretching my mouth wide, split-end hunting, repeating words under my breath, skin-picking—each a ritual of relief, an attempt to siphon off the angst. When my needs aren't met, I don't demand. I don't fight. I shrink. Eric channels our parents' marital stress into roughhousing, his clobbering landing squarely on me. I learn quickly that yelling doesn't summon rescue—it only adds to the noise. His teenage friends work out their sexual curiosities on me and I learn it's better to disappear while their groins insist my leg is a scratching post. The only time I use my voice is when I'm not pinned down, when I'm not rendered physically helpless. When the babysitter—wrapped in a white bath towel after a dip on the hot tub—gets an erection and asks me to sit on his lap, I calmly tell him "No" and go back to playing with my dolls as if he's offered me a PB&J. The next day while mom showers, I casually recount the details through a steamy, glass door. Irate and still dripping wet, she marches next door to confront his mother. I don't think much of this event. The image of the white tent between my sitter's legs files itself in my brain's *That was weird!* Box—because, for once, I had a choice. And I said *no*.

The anxious, repetitive tics, however, are sorting through other boxes—the ones I've hidden even from myself. My body remembers what my mind has long buried. My throat yells and my needs become known every time I silently stretch my mouth. My arms shove boys' bodies away every time I squeeze my shoulders. I extract a thimbleful of longing every time I pop a pimple. These behaviors soothe but also control me. The family jokes about *Kimmy's weird tics,* and I'm none the wiser. My body speaks in the only language it has left.

Ballet channels this tendency. Obsessing over perfect extensions, perfect turn-out, perfect arches, perfect fouteés keeps me from surfacing that which I'd sooner destroy. But ballet is more than an outlet for my anxious wiring. The dance studio becomes my church. The dancers, my congregation. I feel whole when I'm with them, training, rehearsing, performing. Our bond is born from sticky sweat, bloody toes, smelly dance bags and thousands of hours bending our bodies toward an impossible ideal. I call us friends but we are more than this. We are sisters. We live for the belief that each day, we will be a bit better than the last.

Our bodies hurt all the time and we welcome it. Our pain becomes our joy.

CHAPTER 7

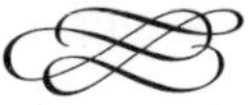

Appleton is different from Kaukauna, the small paper mill town where I spent my elementary years with Jenny. Appleton is bigger, busier. It's the portrait of conservative Midwest except for Lawrence University, an island of progressive ideas, at its center.

Kaukauna was where rural kids went to school, and it's where I learned the unspoken rules of fitting in, the quiet negotiations of childhood friendships. *Be extra nice to everyone. Don't flaunt your grades. Never tell classmates that Dad is a doctor. Make sure Mom picks you up a block away from school so kid's don't see you crawl into her red Audi. Don't do anything to stand out. Don't wear anything to stand out. Lie about the locale of family vacations. At birthday gatherings, make sure your gift is nice, but not* <u>*too*</u> *nice. Be cautious with inviting peers to the house.*

One time I got up the guts to invite some new friends to my fourth-grade birthday party. Later that day, on the bus ride home, I found a hand written note wedged between the seat cushions: "Are you going to Kim Warner's birthday? I'm not. I don't want to go to that rich bitch's house." I don't remember much about my party but I will never forget that note.

Am I a bitch? Shy, yes. But I study my "finishing school" etiquette with diligence. I prioritize the comfort of my peers over my own. I like school, I do my homework, I love PE and recess, but at school everything is underscored by the impossible task of making sure everyone thinks I'm the sweetest thing since Fun Dip Candy Sticks. *Maybe she has money, but she makes up for it in spades because "Boy that Kim, she's so thoughtful, she's so sweet.* And what is being thoughtful, sweet, generous, and kind supposed to buy me in my imaginary plot with the universe? A sense of belonging.

I long to belong.

But am I okay with my longing? That's decades away. The belly ache of yen goes where all the unwanted feelings go—my personal emotional trash compactor. *Get small, get quiet, go numb. If I don't feel the feeling, maybe it won't exist.* Had I let it stay—had I allowed longing to stretch its legs, breathe—I might've seen the irony of acceptance. When I can *be* with my longing, I *be*long. Maybe not to everywhere, not to everyone, but to my body, my truth, myself.

So when Mom and Dad decide to send me to junior high in Appleton, I am relieved to meet classmates who don't judge me for the money my parents make. It's like walking onto a new planet. Girls experiment with their clothes, actually *trying* to stand out. Guys think it's cool that Dad works at the hospital up the street. The social strata is much more diverse and I sense that there is room for me, whatever that means.

During my first PE class, we are summoned into the girls' locker room for a routine scoliosis test. I know the term—one of my ballet friends wears a plastic torso brace for it—but beyond that, I haven't given it much thought.

Mrs. Funk instructs us to line up along the gym lockers and bend forward while removing our shirts. I don't know what the other girls are thinking, but to me, this feels like an awfully intimate introduction to my new classmates. But I oblige. Bow. Shirt off. Exposed.

It's only when I stand upright that my face begins to burn, and not from the blood that pooled in my upside-down skull. I am the only girl without a bra. It hadn't occurred to me that girls wear bras, even if you're still built like a boy. It's just protocol once you're in junior high? An awful layer of satin or lace under my tee shirt? I cringe at the idea of wearing one and I'm horrified at the idea of not. I don't remember anyone being particularly mean about my naiveté that day but I also have a really good delete button in my brain for the more traumatic events of life. Needless to say, that night Mom takes me to Marshall Fields lingerie department. We buy a white, mesh athletic bra and I wear the same one for years.

My boobs don't make an appearance until well into my twenties, so my seventh-grade initiation into puberty—or lack thereof—etches an obsessive thought pattern into my brain. Later, this synapse will be rewired, replaced with an ever-growing list of obsessive, intrusive thoughts and magical thinking loops. But for a good five to six years all I want are boobs—if I do chest exercises I'll get boobs, if I eat chicken, I'll get boobs, if I think the right thoughts, I'll get boobs. Eventually, when I'm eighteen, I ask Dad (who had recently read a book about hypnotherapy) if he could hypnotize me and help my boobs grow. Boundaries anyone? I think the appropriate response from a father should have been, "No." Or "How about I find you a qualified hypnotherapist?" Or even better "Let's find something more constructive for you to worry about!" But instead, he says "Sure."

We head to the meditation room. Of course. I sit cross legged by the window and he sits across the room assuming his objective but kindly physician's demeanor. I feel terribly awkward but his clinical approach puts me at ease. Somewhat. He doesn't say "boob." He says "breast tissue." As if that makes it all okay.

What follows is a pretty uneventful trip down some stairs, counting backwards as I descend. When I reach *one* I am still completely aware of the room, the Saturday afternoon sun blazing across my legs, the hot itch I feel in my chest when something is shoved unconsciously into my emotional trash compactor. Besides wanting our experiment to work, I want Dad to feel like he's doing a good job. I fake my way through it and later retell the experience as a funny (yet failed) hypnotherapy session. Padded bra sales at Marshall Fields go up that season.

As with the botched toe-stubbing experiment, I convince myself that Dad's hypnosis failed because *I* failed, because my mind is flawed. *If I could just control my thoughts, everything would fall into place.*

* * *

My ballet buddy Corinne and I write motivational quotes on our hands throughout high school—daily reminders of how to be better. And there's no harm in a little self-improvement. We can all benefit from self-reflection, examining our conditioning, setting goals. But for me, this pattern of thinking isn't just a practice; it's a lifeline. Or rather, an anti-lifeline.

Obsessive thinking pulls me further and further from the discomfort of simply existing. If I just think the right thought, eat the right food, master the right technique, take the right herb—my boobs will grow, my pimples will disappear, my fouettés will be perfect, my body will be pain-free, my heart will be happy. If I can control my mind, I can control my body. The unpredictable mystery of flesh is not allowed off-leash. This kind of thinking haunts me. The illusion of control is my narcotic of choice over acceptance—I don't want to *be* myself. I want to *fix* myself.

I toggle between total detachment and riding the high of perfection. The chase continues to ignite me, kindling aliveness. And yet. The chase inevitably ends and numbness returns waiting for its next challenge. The circle of life, but different.

On the surface, the Warners are the perfect family. Handsome doctor husband; educated and career-woman wife with the cheekbones of Cindy Crawford; popular, life-of-the-party teenage son; ballerina, straight-A student daughter. We have social circles, spiritual circles, and creative circles—men's groups, women's groups, wellness groups, goddess groups, mother-daughter groups. We have deep conversations. We talk about our feelings. We even meditate together facing the four directions associated with our birthdays—a harmonious circle of East, West, North and South. What a pretty picture. But look closely.

The compass needle is broken. Dad's true north is different than Mom's. Eric's points toward his friends. Mine wavers somewhere between people-pleasing and solitude and longing—sometimes by choice, mostly by default. I am home alone a lot. Evenings blur into an endless loop of sitcoms and bowls of Grape Nuts. If I hear someone in the driveway, I duck behind the kitchen island. A recurring nightmare haunts me—two strange men idling in a '59 Chevy convertible, lurking, loitering, waiting. I dull my fear under the weight of held breath.

But when I'm with others, I become something else entirely—my compass spinning, recalibrating, hypersensitive to the magnetic pull of other people's needs. It never quite lands. And so I retreat to solitude—not a peaceful kind, but an aloneness that lingers, unmoved by neither presence or absence.

I ground myself with routine, structure and predictability. Mom is thoughtful about our activities, maintaining our calendar even through the more tumultuous stretches of her marriage. She may need the predictability as much as I do. Holiday rituals, meal rituals, Kim Robertson's calming harp-music-in-the-morning rituals. The structure soothes my nervous system, but the confidence with which it's executed sedates me. I fall in line. Who am I to question these three gorgeous, intelligent, successful humans and the way they move so assuredly through the world?

I don't have the language or confidence to explore my own unasked, unanswered questions. Ask me if something is wrong and I feel a) guilty feeling like shit when I have so much privilege b) confused by the disconnect between how I feel and how I am perceived c) grumpy and embarrassed when you notice that I feel like shit and d) sad when you don't notice that I feel like shit.

And this is when I take it out on myself, on my skin. I spend hundreds of hours hidden in the bathroom, punishing myself, excavating anxiety one pore at a time. Blood and sebum surface like proof. I don't understand the source of my unease, so I create one instead. *The root of my anxiety must be my skin.* Why would I think otherwise? There is nothing in the outward-facing architecture of my life that explains why I feel like an outsider—so lonely, so deeply insecure. So I latch onto the one thing I can see. If only these pimples go away, then I'll be happy again. I am soothed by the hypnotic, obsessive, compulsive scrutinizing, squeezing and picking. But after each session, I emerge, face-inflamed.

Deep down, I want nothing more than to be held and witnessed in my mess, I squeeze chaos to the surface for its chance to be met with unconditional love. But instead, I cancel plans with friends, I forgo a goodnight hug from Mom or Dad, dating is out of the question—I can't possibly imagine kissing a boy until someone invents a smudge-free, tsunami-proof cover-up. Intimacy means I have to show my face, my true face, and I'm quite certain I have no idea who that is anyway. I'm not ready to be seen in my vulnerability and if I play that one forward, I only see rejection—not so much rejection by others but a complete annihilation and rejection of myself. So instead, I b-line it to my dark bedroom and plea to the universe to heal my skin. That will fix everything.

SEPTEMBER 1, 1992

Dear Charlie,

Today something strange happened.

When I got home from school Mom asked me to go for a walk with her. We never go for walks together. She joined the jogging movement in the 80's so I occasionally run alongside her while she pounds marital stress out through her feet. But a leisurely, springtime jaunt? I was suspicious.

She began by saying, "This is Dad's idea, not mine."

We set out onto State Park Road under overcast skies. The lake flies were beginning their autumn hatch so the air hummed with a green, high-pitched stench. Mom had one of her marriage and family counselor hats on—her statements felt rehearsed and a bit too conclusive. She's very convincing in this state and I find it easy to not question what I hear. Why would I? Her presentation is complete, as if the gods have already brought everything to trial and she is simply reporting the golden truth. She means well. She loves fiercely, generously, wants only the best for me. But sometimes through her clear, resonant note of positivity, I hear something else. It's faint and usually fades quickly. I heard it today. For a fraction of a second, I felt like I was remembering a sequence of notes from a dream and if I could just hold on a bit longer, I'd recall the entire melody.

Mom turned to me and stated plainly, "There is a chance that Dad isn't your biological father,"—I HEAR THE NOTE!—"but isn't it more inter-

esting to know now that you belong to the mystery?"—AND NOW IT'S GONE.

I don't know about you but when I receive emotionally loaded news wrapped inside someone's opinion, I take refuge in certainty. If the opinion is plausible, if I respect the person, it's so much easier to adopt their belief in the moment and sort out my feelings later.

Mom needed a beautiful, happy story. So I did too.

Her conviction was clear and sunny, and much more preferable to the hairline fracture forming inside me, threatening to crack open and obliterate everything.

Yes Mom, the mystery. That sounds good.

CHAPTER 8

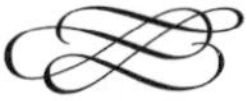

Later in life Mom and I will debate my response. She remembers that *I* was the one who concluded, "So this must mean I belong to the mystery." I don't remember this at all, but I also don't remember some significant chunks from childhood, especially some of the more emotionally loaded ones. *The delete button*. Maybe Mom is right. Maybe I did say something about belonging to the mystery. But if I did, I said it for her. It's so much more beautiful, more poetic, to be a daughter of the mystery than a daughter of a stranger.

The invisible tentacles of my mind had already had seventeen years of practice reaching into the dark boxes of other people's heads and figuring out how they wanted me to respond. It's much safer to fit myself into another person's truth than tug on the thread of my own—because if I did, my story might unravel. My sense of being an outsider would no longer be a *sense*, it would be a truth.

Did I know deep in my bones that I was "different", that I wasn't a Warner?

Did I push that intuition away by denying myself a voice, afraid that if I spoke up, the dissonance would be alarmingly clear?

. . .

I want nothing more than to fit in with my family, especially to be accepted by Mom and Dad. And not because I feel like they're the "cool crowd" and I admire all their qualities; rather, I'm terrified of my own truth and the consequences of it surfacing. So, my teenage brain receives the paternity uncertainty as *odd* and I dismiss it. *Delete. Backspace. Move to Trash.* I put that "beautiful, happy story" away. I never bring it up with Dad. I never share the story with friends. I don't even remember turning it over in my own mind.

Mom had presented the paternity question as a "low possibility" going as far to explain that if I were Charlie's daughter, I would have been born premature. I was small at birth but not premature; I was considered healthy. *See? No reason to question.*

Besides, Dad and I have such a strong bond. All my life Mom has claimed I have his lower lip. His legs. His affinity for math and science. Dad's parents once wondered where I got my nose and then traced it back to a paternal great aunt.

I think about how Dad, in the quiet of my infancy, once let the question flicker in his mind—*Is she mine?* But the thought unsettled him. Afraid I could "psychically" hear him, he pushed it away, made a promise to himself in that moment: *I will always believe she is my daughter. She is my daughter.*

Mom doesn't remember Charlie's full name "His last name is maybe Bower, Bowerman, Brewer" she says, grasping at syllables lost in time. DNA tests aren't yet easily accessible, nor the *Information Super Highway.*

So, with no evidence to the contrary, I take what I've been given—the only dad I know.

My Dad.

I'll take him. I'll keep him.

* * *

That winter I enroll in a senior year "blow off" class called Interpersonal. I first heard about it as a sophomore and imagined all the seniors—finally carefree and wise—sitting in a circle and sharing feelings for a grade. Mrs. Haack, who also teaches English, runs the class with an attentiveness that flourishes here in a way it never quite can in a standard lit curriculum. We journal. We write letters to each other. We examine and challenge our belief systems, our choices, our dreams. In the thick of senior year—the relentless grind of college applications, the mounting pressure to map out a future—this class slows us down. Mrs. Haack coaxes us out of the race and back into ourselves, into each other.

Mrs. Haack gives our parents an assignment, too: *write a letter to your almost-graduate, something meaningful, something hard to say out loud.* She collects these letters, seals them, and promises to mail them to us, unopened, one year later. Dad takes on this assignment with his usual demonstrative love. Along with his letter to me, he makes a mix tape with his favorite dance music. Lately he's been trying to combat depression with morning movement sessions in the basement before heading to the hospital. He stops his Zoloft prescription because "it takes away his dreams."

I hear the tunes pulsing through the kitchen floor as I eat breakfast—slightly embarrassed and yet endeared. While my friends have dads who wake up with coffee, mine greets the day by shaking his pelvis to the hypnotic drumming of Gabrielle Roth.

After school that day, Dad picks me up in his new Volvo. He kept his old vanity plate so the familiar word YANG slowly approaches the curb.

Just a week earlier, we road-tripped to Milwaukee to hunt for a prom dress—more an excuse for a dad-daughter day than a love for shopping (or prom)—but I like that he's game for the adventure. Post-Cinnabon sugar high and mall frenzy, he felt sleepy so I hopped behind the wheel and drove us home. He was fast asleep as I navigated through the small farming towns in central Wisconsin—a sea of wheat and corn interrupted by the occasional one-church, one-bar township. Occasionally I glanced at Dad. His head leaned awkwardly against the window, his jaw slack. Sleep and death wear the same face.

Now, he sits in the driver's seat and I can't shake that image of him from a week ago. As I buckle my seatbelt, I notice he's quieter than usual and doesn't hit the gas right away. With the car idling, I look at him. He's wearing a pale pink, button down shirt. His hair is pulled into a low, tight pony-tail. He smells good. He always smells good. Rubbing alcohol, ylang ylang and something earthy that is uniquely *Dad*. His face is tired as he reaches his right hand to his chest and says "My heart hurts today."

I don't know what this means exactly, but it makes mine ache too. Tangling my feelings up with Dad's is second nature. He always carries a heaviness, but today, it unsettles me. I don't reply in words. Instead, my heart mirrors his weight, my own ache folding into his, and burrowing deep into the quiet chambers of my chest.

* * *

Friday comes. April 2nd 1993. I get home late. Dad's still out, at some work party. Mom's asleep. The house is silent, save for our beloved mutt Raisin, who shuffles around and lifts her head in mild acknowledgment before settling back down. I'm exhausted from training for a new waitress job, and tomorrow can't come soon enough. I collapse onto my bed, knowing the alarm will pull me out of sleep far too soon. In just a few hours, Mom, Dad, and I will be heading to the airport to catch our flight to Mexico for spring break. Eric, in his second year at the University of Colorado Boulder, will fly separately and meet us there.

No wine spills on anyone's lap my first night of waitressing, so I drift off feeling a small sense of accomplishment—and a bigger sense of anticipation for warm sun and turquoise blue water.

But these things never come.

* * *

"He'll have to drive himself to the airport," Mom says…I wish I could say I'd felt something, noticed a bird soaring outside our gate's window. Saw a child and father embrace near the Apple Vacations ticketing counter. Something. Anything to mark the moment when, at 5:43am, Dad drove head first into a truck—his soul breaking free from the jaws of life just a half hour behind us on Highway 43, racing to make the flight. The insignificant little town of Fredonia cradled his crushed ribs that morning as his spirit unfurled its tireless wings. Or maybe they were tired. I don't know.

* * *

Dear Charlie…

PART II
POLARITY

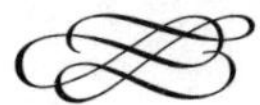

CHAPTER 1

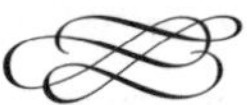

On Easter Sunday, one week after the accident, First Congregational Church holds a memorial for Dad. I wake up that morning to more fat snowflakes. I slip into a long grey skirt and a pair of Bjorn clogs, wondering if they're appropriate. But then, what is? I don't have a map for grief. Mom encourages Eric and me to speak at the memorial, so I shove a Valentine's Day card—one I wrote for Dad, still resting on his side of the bathroom vanity—into my jacket pocket. If I can work up the courage, I will read it out loud.

I walk to the front door of the church with Mom and Eric. Red tulips lining the path, each one crowned in a winter-white hat. Dad loved a good paradox; this stark juxtaposition of seasons would've made him smile. Death and rebirth? Check. A memorial service on Easter Sunday? Check. Deviled eggs and angel food cake at the repast? Check.

I feel eyes on us as we walk to the front of the congregation and take a seat. The sanctuary is large but fills quickly—winter jackets and warm bodies pressing in. Before the memorial begins I glance behind me. Dad touched so many lives; there is standing room only. Friends and acquaintances spill into the foyer like a black river, rising, ready to pull me under.

Our musician friends, Patty and Larry, take the stage and begin playing *Wings*—a song they composed in the wake of Dad's sudden death. As the first notes rise, my gaze drifts to the towering bird-of-paradise bouquets. I beseech the blood-orange petals to give me flight. There are drums. Loud drums. The percussion shudders through my chest, cracking the iceberg lodged beneath my ribs. Goosebumps lift across my skin and threaten my unravelling.

Later, I'll learn I wasn't the only one gutted by the music. A letter will arrive from an anonymous community member who, moved by news of a local surgeon's tragic death, decided to attend. Wheelchair-bound, he writes that during the song, he was certain he could fly.

Dad's younger brother rises to speak. He walks to the podium and takes a long, commanding pause. When he finally speaks, his voice is steady. Deliberate.

"The day I learned of my big brother's death, the sky was bruised purple-gray. I went outside to watch the storm roll in, trying to comprehend the impossible. And then I spoke directly to the sky."

"David."

His voice resonates into the microphone, somber and certain. But there's no answer.

He calls again, louder, looking directly at the congregation. We are the storm cloud and somewhere within in it is his big brother.

"David."

Still nothing. It's still not loud enough. Not for his big brother.

"David!" The microphone whistles with the force of his plea. But still, no reply.

He shoves the microphone aside, grips the podium. And then, with his whole body, his whole breaking heart, he tries one last time.

"DAAAAAAAAVVVVVVVIIIIIIIIIIIIIDDDDDD."

The microphone wails, a deafening shriek crashing into the walls, the ceiling, my stopped heart.

No reply.

No one dares move. No one breathes. We wait.

I am shaking, aching to wail in return, desperate to hear Dad wail back. But the silence holds.

Then come the sniffles. Stifled whimpers. We can no longer

suppress grief under a posture of *appropriateness*. What is appropriate when someone you love has just died? Dad's brother broke the dam in all of us. Our soft, animal bodies awaken from shock and feel what is incomprehensible to feel. Death is always incomprehensible. One minute someone is here, the next, they aren't.

But in this moment, I am certain of one thing—Dad is here. His giant, loving presence is called into the room through our communion. We listen for him. We hold space for his reply. And while we hear nothing, we most definitely feel him—shaking his liberated Gabrielle Roth hips in every one of our bruised hearts.

My uncle's gutted offering gives me courage to speak, so long as Eric stands by my side. I don't remember what I say—Do I read the Valentine's card? Do I cry?— but I can recall the warmth of my big brother's presence beside me. He is suffering in his own way. We share the loss but the grief is vastly different. I will never be able to completely reach outside of my own story of grief to understand his. But we stand aside each other and fumble our way through this unexpected union. For Dad.

When the two-and-a-half hour memorial is over, we walk out to the foyer. Classmates I never thought would care stand in a receiving line. Football players, skaters, cheerleaders—the whole *Breakfast Club* of students—are here for me, for my family. Their presence, their warmth, surprises me. Moves me.

I step away from Mom and Eric when I spot them—my ballet sisters, huddled in the corner like a sanctuary. Juanita Makaroff, our fierce and unyielding teacher, stands among them. But today, her face is different. The sharp edges of discipline have softened, the strict ballet master dissolving into something quieter. A motherly protectress. She opens her arms and I fall in. My friends follow, piling their bodies into the warmth. A circle of long, graceful arms embrace me for a safe, comforting eternity.

* * *

But eternity is a misnomer; eternity doesn't last. The circle loosens, and I step back into the world—one that keeps moving, indifferent to the weight pressing down on me. The days blur. I float through them, barely touching solid ground.

As valedictorian, I am asked to give a graduation speech but somehow I get out of it. My brain turns to oatmeal after Dad's death. Is it the cold medicine I take for a cough—and then a little longer—that pleasantly numbs my senses? I drift through the final weeks of high school barely there. A thick, black gauze tangles itself around my body. I start slamming doors; a hinged finality briefly startling me back to life.

Shortly after the memorial, Dad's body is sent to the crematorium. One of his close psychiatrist friends—who Mom not so affectionately calls "Luke the Kook"—suggests we visit his body before the cremation. None of us do. The police report—*steering wheel lodged into his ribcage*—paints a clear enough picture for me. The day after his cremation the local newspaper reports that the Paper Valley Crematorium has caught fire.

I fantasize that when Dad's soul was released from its 49 year-old home, it burst forth with such magnificence that the hot, brick oven couldn't contain it. That he broke free, incinerating the walls that tried to hold him. He escaped the confines of mortal life with one hearty, flagrant roar— a motorcycle rider leaning into the wind, full throttle.

On prom night, I slip into Dad's leather jacket searching for my own roar. I need this weight and scent on me. I will wear this with my prom dress. It will look perfect; well, no it might not, but it will feel perfect. I will feel.

Standing in a friend's backyard along the Fox River, I pose for prom photos in a sequined polka-dot dress, swallowed in his black, wide-shouldered cowhide, and find a pack of half-smoked Marlboro Reds in the inside zip-pocket. *Wait, Dad smoked?* I thought he had one rebellious moment with a cigarette a decade ago, but his biker identity was elusive to all of us so I shouldn't be surprised.

When the parent's are done snapping photos my friends and I walk to the river. I pull out the pack from Dad's jacket, happy to share his secret with my friends.

“Oh you bad boy Dave,” my friend Ana says as she reaches into the crumpled pack. I wonder how much time has passed since his fingers grazed these white tips. I have a sudden impulse to hold every cigarette in my hands. I want to press them to my cheek, shove them in my mouth, make whatever is left of Dad a part of me.

While my imagination devours a tobacco buffet, my friends light up and one by one, quietly take a little bit of David Warner into their lungs.

“To Dave,” they say, exhaling him into the late spring breeze. He twirls easily into nothingness while my lungs try to hold him near. I sit on the edge of the river bank letting the smoke warm my mostly-virgin bronchi and watch my friends. The way they pass the cigarette with quiet reverence, the way they speak his name like a prayer. I am overwhelmed by their kindness, their sincerity. Turns out, sharing time, puberty and cheap beer can forge something greater—something that shows up when it matters most.

The morning of graduation a few friends go fishing and catch a foot-long carp. Naturally, they bring it to the ceremony, swaddled in a few layers of Saran Wrap. As the procession of students winds toward the podium to receive diplomas, a fish arcs above a river of black caps as if jumping for flies. I walk up, accept my diploma and sit back down with the same enthusiasm as taking out the trash. The empty chair beside Mom renders the ceremony a hollow formality. My heart feels like that fish—gutted, out of place, gasping for something that isn’t there. So to see this dead carp flopping in the middle of it all, I almost laugh. Of course. Of course, a lifeless thing, lost and absurd, would be the only thing that makes sense.

CHAPTER 2

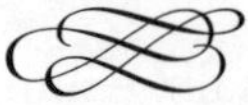

SUMMER BEGINS. Day's stretch wide and empty, the kind of summer that should be filled with dance, swimming and long afternoons with friends. But this isn't a typical summer. I spend most days alone, poring over condolence letters, writing in my journal, wandering aimlessly through the house. A hazy escape from reality might lend itself well to more time at the ballet barre but instead I feel shaky and weak and often exit class before center adagio.

Mom encourages me to go to therapy to "work with my grief." It will take decades to realize why talk therapy rarely leads to breakthroughs for me. Chalk it up to my reflexive ability to sense what people want to hear, what will appease them, what will make them feel good about themselves. Therapy is just another place for me to ensure my shrink is sleeping well at night.

You want me to cry? Ok, here are some tears. You want me to write a letter to my dead dad? Sure, let me pour out some poetic sorrow. You want me to breathe into the achy bits and tell you what they say? They are sad. Right? And angry. Yes, of course. Angry. You want me to make a sound with that anger? Rar! My breakthroughs are cashed in at $80 a session but the only one losing sleep is me.

I am also losing a grip on reality through magical thinking. In my journals, I talk to Dad as if he never left. Late afternoons, I sit at the edge of the dock, watching the golden sun glint off the water and convincing myself it's him—his energy, his presence, shimmering around me wherever I go. I start distrusting my senses, deciding my eyes are the ones lying to me. *Even though I can't see him, Dad is most certainly, most definitively, right next to me.* It's a comforting lie, one I cradle tightly, a suffocating blanket over the rage and confusion I refuse to let surface. Magical thinking lives up to its name. The moment an unwelcome emotion arrives, I shape-shift it into a happy ending. *Dad's gone* becomes *He's free from his physical form. He's even closer to me. He's with me all the time.* The vast mystery of death—of existence itself—shrinks to a certainty I can hold. A story I can live with.

But even Mom can't hold this one, not all the time. One night I lay awake in bed, the window wide open. The gentle lapping of water on shore drifts in, a rhythmic hush against the night. Moonlight spills across my room, casting blue shadows over the dance posters on my wall. The house is hushed except for familiar pops and creaks of shifting logs and rafters. But there's something more —a sound I'm not accustomed to hearing. Is it coming from outside? A red fox and her cubs yipping in the trees? I get up to investigate. Leaving my room, I tiptoe silently as if it's the only polite way to walk amongst sleeping giants.

When I reach the loft, I kneel at the railing overlooking the family room below. Everything is illuminated by moonlight and Mom sits in the middle of it. The old, black rocking chair shifts under her weight. It has been in the family for as long as I can remember. Usually draped with a sheep skin rug, this was Dad's favorite place to sit and read Anne Rice novels or watch Star Trek. However, I don't ever remember Mom sitting in it, much less *sitting*. Tonight, her body and the chair are one shape, turned inside out by the sound that escapes from it. I have never in eighteen years seen—or heard—Mom cry like this. Anguished sobs fall out of her like hail.

I only remember her crying one other time. I was in the third grade and I came home to find her sitting on the sofa (unusual) watching *Little House On the Prairie* (even more unusual), silent tears rolling down her cheeks.

Tonight, her wails echo throughout the house and land in my chest. I don't know how such tortured sadness can simultaneously feel reverent, but it does. In this moment, I am certain that even through all the tumultuous chapters of Mom and Dad's life together, it was founded and grounded in a profound—if confusing —love.

Dad's ashes sit in the meditation room for the entire summer. Occasionally I go in, sit cross-legged on the carpeted floor and lift the lid. The tin is heavy. In movies, ashes drift weightlessly, scattering like a spirit finally released on wings of angels. But Dad's ashes are more like gravel—small, white chunks of bone and grit. I sift them between my fingers, expecting something softer. Something light. Couldn't fire, the great alchemist, transform the weight of Dad's depression too?

This isn't wholly how I remember Dad. But I do know he struggled—constantly trying new medications, quitting them because of side-effects, and then starting again. He came home drained from long hours at the hospital, his frustration palpable. His vision for cardiac health was too progressive for a Midwestern hospital in the 1980s. Following a triple bypass surgery, patients were served double cheese burgers and fries. And his stress-management techniques? Pure quackery, as far as the hospital was concerned.

At the same time, one of Dad's favorite quotes was, "Beer and franks with cheer and thanks is better than sprouts and bread with fear and dread." Dad was a living enigma. He was a responsible surgeon and a capricious husband. He devoted his time and intellect to medical sciences, but he also loved his Harley. He revered the complex, mystical mechanics of sentient life but he was reckless with his own. Another favorite quote of his was "Take everything in moderation, including moderation." With a blood alcohol level of .12 at the time of the accident, that one may have killed him.

Dad often said the best part of being a cardiac surgeon was "doing rounds." I proudly walked the hospital corridors by his side —his magnetic, vertically-blessed presence drawing smiles and admiration from staff and patients alike. He would kneel at a patient's bedside to meet them at eye level, his hand resting gently on their forearm. His deep, resonant voice carried reassurance, a salve for healing tissue. This is what he loved most—not just the precision of surgery, but the humanity of care.

The operating room was more mechanical, methodical. As a teen, I watched him perform surgery and nearly lost my lunch while they cut through the torso of a large man, ribcage unfurled to meet Dad's gloved hands. But despite the blood and steel, there was an artistry to it—a strangely beautiful, well-choreographed ballet. Everyone in the room knew their part, their movements precise, their timing impeccable.

And then, the finale. The patient's heart took center stage. Stitches in place and bypass complete, Dad glanced over at me and winked as the technician turned off the cardiopulmonary bypass machine. The room fell silent. Everyone waited. And waited.

Then—a miracle.

The little lump of red and blue flesh, shuddered and wriggled its way back into a beat. Lub dub. Lub dub. Or in dad's medical terminology – *love dub, love dub.*

Summer grief presses a sweaty hand on my back. Lake Winnebago turns from dishwater brown to green to unswimmable so I swim in memories of Dad instead. No, drown in them. My body clenches around grief, an ache with no release.

I close my eyes and remember.

Dad and I are driving down Lake Park Road, music blasting through car speakers. I'm sticky with ballet sweat, he's sticky with depression. We work it out through the music, throwing arms into space, conducting notes into crescendos that pull the tiny hairs on our arms into unison. Sadness, disappointment, muscle ache, heart ache—all are welcome.

I want the music to last forever; the road's long, straight arm reaches into a blackened horizon, then the County Highway 114 intersection. We turn left, hugging the lake at 55mph. We pass Fire Lane 8. Fire Lane 9. Fire Lane 10. Practical emergency routes become imaginary runways for boys and Big Wheels. We pass Fire Lane 13, the stabled horses are steady and heavy-lidded, trading speed for silence while flies keep the balance.

We reach Country Side Bar—fried cheese and smoke fill my senses. Turn right onto State Park Road. Our orchestra becomes fast and furious and our arms rejoice the home stretch. But just as my stomach gurgles and my mind fixates on a bowl of cereal, Dad abandons course. A secret, mischievous minuet inside his chest needs air. There is no right turn, but he takes it anyway. The cows see grass for grazing, he sees a runway for flying. Farmer Don Mielke looks up from his newspaper, startled by headlights blasting through his pasture, but then dismisses it as the onset of a migraine. Windows down, the tall grass throws a fist-full of life into my nose. Dad laughs out loud and throws a fist-full of love into my heart.

He slows down when we reach the other side of the field, finding a shallow ditch to navigate us safely back to concrete. He turns off the ignition but my mind is ignited with sensation, with freedom. In my imagination, we are still driving. No, flying. In the damp, oily stench of the garage we listen to the hypnogogic clicks of the engine. One machine and two time-keeping muscles are joined in the dream state. One longer click. One shorter one. One longer, one shorter. Lub dub, lub dub.

Love dub, love dub.

CHAPTER 3

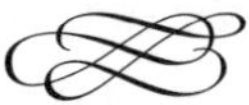

The insignificant little town of Fredonia cradled his crushed ribs that morning as his spirit unfurled its tireless wings. Or maybe they were tired. I don't know.

Mom deconstructs the word—Fredonia—and reimagines it as Fré Donné—free the woman. Eric and I latch onto this, a powerful fragment of the story, maybe even a message from Dad beyond the grave. Was it his final wish for her? To free her from the endless cycles of betrayal and reconciliation? In this small, unremarkable town, a secret to Dad's salvation reveals itself, offering us a lifeline of meaning. We cling to it, desperate for consolation, for some proof that his death wasn't just an accident on a lonely stretch of road, but part of a larger, unseen design.

I look into the etymology now and can't find anything that says that Fré means "free"; instead, I read that it originates from Old French *freid* from Latin *frigidus.* It doesn't mean "free." It means "cold." Cold woman?

Cold Woman or Free the Woman. I laugh out loud. Which narrative would *you* choose?

. . .

Just weeks before I pack up the maroon mini-van and drive west to Colorado College (cool-dom here I come?), Mom, Eric and I decide it's time to release Dad's ashes—on her 49th birthday.

We gather fallen branches and yard debris, dragging them to the rocky shoreline below our house. Eric helps us stack the pile as high as his head—a funeral pyre fit for the gods. At sundown, he douses it in gasoline, tosses a match, and flames lick the last light in the sky. Bonfires are a favorite summer ritual, a way to clear out the season's remnants—branches, deadwood, shoreline debris. But tonight there are no marshmallows, no beer. None of us really know how to do this, how to send a body back to the elements, how to mark the end of a life with fire. But somber feels right, so we let it be.

While sparks dance around our heads, we drag a mostly-neglected canoe onto the rocks and into shallow water. Mom wanted this canoe for her 40th birthday, imagining countless, Orangesicle-sky evenings where she and Dad would paddle deep into Winnebago's quiet. These purchases rarely mirror the fantasy. I can count on one hand the times we actually hauled it out, always favoring the ease and weightlessness of flailing limbs careening off the end of the dock.

Tonight, we are glad to have something to haul. The dead weight of it pressing down on our shoulders is right. Tonight, this ancient shape will carry us, and what's left of Dad, into the rippling shadows of Winnebago. As we paddle away from shore, the textures beneath us shape shift from flickering, vibrant orange, to creamsicle pink, purple, and eventually black.

When we are well past the sand bars and certain that Dad's ashes won't wash up on our neighbor's shore, we lay down our oars and let the canoe rock. Mom in the stern, Eric in the bow, me in the middle. The bonfire is a distant, pulsing ember—our only tether to land, our navigation home. We sit for a long time in silence, letting the canoe drift and sway. The lake is so still that we could sit here all night, suspended between water and sky, never drifting back to shore. Below us, prehistoric sturgeon prowl the depths, their scaleless bodies gliding through the dark, wondering about the shifting black shadow above them. Dad's remains won't be the tasty snack they anticipate. I am haunted by these giant fish. The word *fish* hardly describes their alien presence. Aqua Dinosaur? Limbless Water Torso? In winter months, when the lake freezes solid, ice fisherman drive onto its surface, set up shanties around gaping 4x4 holes and wait. Spears and beer are requisite. Every spring, at least one of their vehicles doesn't make it off in time and becomes curious architecture for bottom dwellers.

I hear the crinkling of a plastic bag as Mom lifts Dad's ashes from his cookie-tin home. We didn't put him in there. He arrived from the crematorium this way. It will forever be the most absurd association I have with death—buttery English biscuits and Dad's crushed bones.

Mom puts on her therapist hat, doing her best to help us navigate the unnavigable. "Let's each share something about Dad," she suggests gently. "A quality of his you'll always carry with you."

I comply, but only because that's what I do. Complying is my nature. My own way of grieving lurks somewhere at the bottom of the lake with the sturgeon, and I don't dare go near this uncharted territory.

Eric takes to the assignment with sacred gusto, scooping a handful of ashes and scattering them over the water. Then, with a quiet reverence, he holds back a final pinch and lifts it to his mouth.

"Eric—" I start, but he's already swallowed.

"He's part of me now," he says simply.

How can I beat that?

Are there tears on the canoe ride? I don't remember. Nor do I remember the qualities of Dad we promise to keep alive. Does it feel strangely ordinary? Or completely surreal? I lean toward the banal in memory, thinking I should be feeling more but I am, again, mostly numb. I go through the *motions* of grief but not the feelings. I am a kid again stubbing my toe around the perimeter of the house. I concluded a decade ago that pain hurts and now I'm getting a real, moment-by-moment opportunity to feel the stabbing in my heart and let it be okay—to feel its intensity and not run. But it's too much. Instead I shove it into the familiar glacial mass in my belly where it is always winter. I join the sturgeon under the ice and avoid the spear at all costs.

Heading to school two weeks later is probably not the best idea.

But the plan is already in place and I'm functioning on autopilot. The highway exit to Colorado College is 143, and so is my freshman dorm room number. I take them as a sign: I'm meant to live out Dad's destiny. Within the first month, I declare my major—Biology/Pre-Med. *If I become a doctor, I will be close to Dad, keep him alive. He will live through me. I will take his DNA's coding and carry it forward, completing what he couldn't. He will talk to me. He will guide me at every turn because I have chosen his path.*

I don't belong to the mystery, I belong to him.

Freshman year is a hazy blur. I stalk a classmate when I learn at orientation that he, too, has lost a parent and I loiter in his dorm room with nothing to say. He is always kind—the way you'd be kind to a stray dog with mange—letting me sit on his bed while he and his buddies smoke weed and listen to Chemical Brothers. My presence puzzles him. I don't want to smoke, I don't want to drink, I don't want to make out. I just want to sit near someone who maybe, just maybe, can sense the life inside me, trapped beneath all this silence, waiting for its chance to surface.

* * *

During winter break, I return to Wisconsin. Familiarity is a comfy old blanket that smells of mold. Dad is still everywhere. Six months is not long enough for our cells to stop reaching. One morning Mom receives a phone call from Mrs. Haack, my high-school Interpersonal teacher. Mom's shoulder cradles the phone as her eyes shift from me, back to the empty space in front of her.

"Yes, I remember," she says as concerned recognition spreads across her face.

Mrs. Haack has a package for me—the 8"x12" padded envelope Dad stuffed twelve months earlier with a typed letter and a mixtape—and wants to make sure it's okay to send. Three days later it arrives in the mailbox. The return address reads: *Dad, You Know Where.*

I rip the padded envelope open with such force that I tear

straight through his letter. A gash through his words, through time itself. Tape mends but cannot untear.

My hands tremble as Dad's words fall into me.

October 16, 1992

Dear Kim,

With all the notes and letters that we have written to each other, this doesn't seem like it is something new. However, the request that it be some of the things where the moment never seems right to say kind of puts it into a different category. Some things pop into mind that I could write about but I'm not sure that they are very important to you; you know, phases that have come cycling by over the last twenty years or so. Stuff that has been impacting on me and seems like it might be important to you, if not on a conscious level, at least at the level of the unconscious stuff that we all have to work with at some time or other. This morning, however, I realized what it was that I mainly wanted to communicate to you. And it came not in the way of words so much as what I was doing at the time; i.e. dancing. And it seems to wrap up a bunch of stuff, so here goes…

There are probably few things in one's life that touch a parent deeper than seeing a family issue being passed on to one's beloved children. This has probably been one of the strongest motivating forces I have encountered. This can apply to the positive ones, I guess; but it seems like the difficult ones, the unconscious stuff that blocks our love from ourselves or someone/thing else, are the ones that often seem to be the most difficult, sometimes ever devastating. I am not such a martyr that I want to take responsibility for all the stuff in the Warner family and maybe even a little of the Larson household. I am learning to love myself too much to do that. And I am enjoying life too much to only focus on the negative aspects of the mostly beautiful hours that I spend each day in relation to my universe of friends, family and the natural world around me. But there is one thing that I think you may have picked up from the Warner family that I have had to work on a great deal and I see that it might become a teacher for you as well. You obviously have a big head start as compared to me at your age (which is the way it is supposed to be) and I am glad of that. Your body-awareness, i.e. your abilities to sense what is going on inside, is really quite remarkable as far as I can see. For me, that journey of exploration has been challenging, although also very rewarding. It has been "my path" in the sense that so much of my learning has come from working out "hang-ups" and trying to find out why certain areas of my body were tighter than others and why vertebrae were starting to mush together.

One of the most exciting and rewarding experiences that I have had was the experience at Esalen when I, for the first time in 40 some years learned what it felt like to really dance. I found the place inside where the dance originates and ways to allow the music to move my body rather than thinking and planning how to do it. I realize that this may be old stuff for you. With your ballet training, I'm sure that you have had to do a lot of that locating already. And I guess that if one is to use the body as a learning tool, he or she would look at what parts are stiff or tight and then go into the energy of that area to see what it had to say to them. We all seem to have some balance to strike between "flowing" or taking things easily on the one hand and discipline or keeping things in control on the other. That sometimes shows up in the way one's body moves (or doesn't move) and where injuries occur. I guess that I am rambling along and may be losing you or you may be wondering what I am really trying to say. Maybe the music can say it better for me. Basically I just wish for you the pleasure and wisdom that comes with letting the dance dance you rather than trying to do it right or the way that it would seem right to others; …the marvelous balance between creating the discipline and then letting go into the flow of the music or the whatever; …the beauty of experiencing the body's unique ability to be an interface between heaven and earth.

With the enclosed tape, what I would suggest is to take about one half of an hour sometime when you can be alone, preferably with room to dance freely, preferably with a sound system that will give you enough quality to hear the words and feel the bass, and then just put the music on and wait. Wait for the music to move you in whatever way that it will. Feel the places in your body that reverberate to the sound and let those areas direct the movement. Particularly the first 30 minutes or so, I like. Anyway, while I was dancing to this, I realized that this really did express so much of what I would like to say to you. My fantasy is that someday you and I will feel comfortable enough with each other that we will put this tape on and dance to it, able to express whatever comes up at the moment and not feel embarrassed or awkward. That is my fantasy and my wish, for I believe that that would mean that both you and I would be in pretty neat places with ourselves (even though we are at this time too, of course.)

Blessings, my darling Kim, and my heart goes with you always.

Love,

Dad

I read it again. And again. I pause to reflect on his words. "I just wish for you the pleasure and wisdom that comes with letting the dance dance you rather than trying to do it right." Sure, I see his point. Ballet has shaped me. Whenever I hear music, I want to spin, point my toes, do *port de bras*. Impulses to wiggle my hips have been conditioned out of me. But why is this *his wish* for me? Of all the wishes a father could have for a daughter, this one confuses me. He wishes that, together, we storm the dancefloor?

I sense he is saying something more but "letting the dance dance me" is treacherous territory. It feeds my magical thinking. It encourages me to side-step reality and develop a growing fascination with the paranormal. *Let the dance dance me.*

I stay up late with my thoughts, with Dad's words. I open up a blank word document on Dad's first generation Apple PowerBook; I will leave it open overnight, the winking cursor will invite his correspondence and surely he'll write me again. I notice it's 1:43 am. As if the number 43 isn't already resonant enough. 143. Shorthand for *I love you.*

I love you, too, Dad. I say it aloud, pleading to see his ghost and fantasizing about becoming a switchboard operator for the deceased.

The following spring semester, I record myself reading his letter, layer it over a track from the mixtape, and choreograph a solo to perform for the living (and conjure the dead). I interpret his wish as prophecy of a literal promise of reunion, completely misunderstanding—or unwilling to brave—his truer longing. *When the setting is right, when the timing is right, when the burning beeswax candle is right, when I'm dancing just right—Dad will return.*

CHAPTER 4

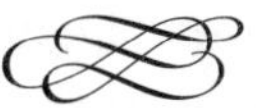

EARLY SOPHOMORE YEAR, I fall in love with Ashton "Ash" Andros. We meet during the first month of Introductory Mandarin Chinese, fatefully paired for a vocabulary exercise. I already had my eyes on him. His lean, athletic build crossing the classroom every morning —skate-board tucked under one arm—my gaze secretly ushering him to his seat.

Today's vocabulary: family members and vocations. We learn how to say, "My mother is an artist." "My father is a businessman." Ignoring the present-tense impossibility of Dad, I turn to my partner—this gorgeous, half-Vietnamese, half-Swiss/Argentinian boyish man—ready to begin the exercise. But instead of playing along, he furrows his dark brow. "Yeah, I'm not into this," he mutters. "My dad's dead."

In a dangerous instant, the doors of my heart are thrown open and Ash walks in.

While the rest of class practices their pronunciation, this stranger and I share stories about our dead fathers. Both, suddenly. Both, tragically—mine from a Mac truck, his from a bad meatball in Bangladesh. Mystery clings to both exits and inflates our fathers' already larger-than-life status.

Life post-Dad and pre-Ash, was an apocalyptic drought. When I meet Ash, a mad thirst awakens in my cells and he is my oasis. We become inseparable. We write letters to our fathers and bury them deep in the foothills of the Rockies. We take ecstasy and scream their disembodied names back into existence. Ash is fearless and passionate because he knows no other way. I flirt with fearlessness and passion because I need his way near.

Our first summer break we road trip to Baja, traveling dirt roads with nothing but tortillas, canned beans, hot sauce, and sharp knives for hunting urchin and scallops in the shallow Sea of Cortez. Pacifico beer, our water. Discarded mattresses on empty beaches, our thrones. At night, the star-studded sky tips upside down and our naked bodies tangle in bioluminescence. At sunrise, we are the last humans watching the only show on earth. We live like a king and queen in a palace of our own making, securing a bond with each other that is born not from two souls, but four.

After a month of adventure, we return to the states so I can spend August with Mom in Wisconsin. I can't conceive of leaving Ash behind, not for a day, much less an entire month, but introducing him to my former life feels scary. Blending worlds is too confusing, too unmooring, for my fragmented identity.

On my way out of town, I park in front of Ash's attic apartment to say goodbye. I pause for a moment and watch him before exiting the car. He sits on the first-floor stoop smoking a cigarette, feet resting on his skateboard. He notices me but his expression doesn't shift; unlike me, Ash's compass needle doesn't waver; he always knowing his true north. I love looking at him. Jet-black hair, burnt-caramel skin. He looks pissed off when he's not smiling. But just under the scowl are deep, boyish dimples that, when offered, make me feel like I'm the only woman in the world.

As I pull away, Earth's female population obliterated, I savor the ash still on my lips.

The sixteen hour drive between Colorado and Wisconsin is long and straight—plenty of spaciousness to allow the feelings of young love to swell into something epic, cinematic. I slide Ash's *Blue Jamaica* mixtape into the car player and with the first notes, I'm back in his room, bathed in the glow of a single blue bulb. Nights stretched endlessly there, time dissolving in the low hum of music and whispered confessions. It was in that room, in the warmth of Ash's attentive desire, that my anatomy shifted from textbook to technicolor.

I turn the volume up. Jimmy Hendrix, Astrud Gilberto, and Miles Davis deliver me back into his arms. A thawing. Tears begin to stream down my face. The paradox of heartache is revealed. Look long and hard enough at it, and suddenly beauty stares back.

AUGUST 3, 1994

Dear Charlie,

You were once in a bar fight, or so I'm told. After finishing your set at a small, rural haunt somewhere in Wisconsin, a drunk patron approached the stage. His girlfriend had been flirting with you. Or maybe you flirted with her? Not one for drama, you dismissed his verbal attack, packed your instruments and walked out to the snowy parking lot. The man was waiting for you.

With your cheek pressed into icy gravel, he kicked you in the gut over and over. Instead of fighting back, you lay there, surrendered to the absurd beauty of it all as snow danced under a single sodium vapor bulb.

I can see it clearly—a few cars, the exterior of a dismal country bar, a single source of light illuminating the scene. One man is painted with rage, the other in blood. The soundtrack, silent. Snowflakes insist on blanketing horror with wonder.

You understand, don't you?

Beauty and pain, such mad lovers.

CHAPTER 9

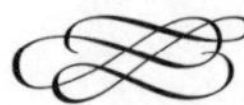

MAD LOVE TENDS NOT to last. I have witnessed this, but now I have lived it. Near the end of my senior year, Ash and I end our relationship. He graduated a year earlier and lives in Crested Butte, skiing backcountry and working as a sushi chef at a small inn. I'm weary of making the four-hour drive, one-way, almost every weekend to visit. It's not the first time we tried ending things, but I'm tired of digesting his reality. I want to taste my own. We have loved each other fiercely, but over time the divide deepens—geographically and otherwise. His temper, my passivity. Almost complementary at first, until it's not.

The summer after graduation, Mom and I visit my grandma in Florida, flying into Miami and then driving at dusk along Alligator Alley—a hot, 80-mile, stretch yawning through the Everglades. Lit only by lampposts and headlights, the looming darkness stirs my own; I begin recounting stories from my three-year relationship with Ash, memories I had tucked away, too ashamed to share—even with myself. Now, I unspool them as if I'm reading aloud someone else's memoir.

Neighbors in a small college town hear shouting and breaking glass. Two young lovers are questioned by police; the woman hides trembling hands, the man hides bloodied hands, with broken glass at their feet. The same young woman sits alone in the hot, Baja desert for a day without money, food or water. When the man returns, her hunger to be powerful is betrayed by her hunger to not be alone. There's a knife. Cornered in a high valley of the Rocky Mountains, the young man points it at his gut as the woman takes the wrong side in an argument. The same woman sleeps in a snow-covered dog house because she'd rather be rescued than rescue herself.

Mom interrupts and asks if I'd like to roll down the window.

"Sure." I say, wondering if she's even listening. "Why?"

"I think you need to scream." She replies, reaching an encouraging hand into mine.

Inhaling, I pull Mom's amber perfume into my lungs, then deeper, where it beckons the cold, lifeless shape in my gut to rise.

At first, thin and timid in my throat. Then warm. Then hot. Then round. Then free. *Fré Donné.*

My smoldering body torches the sky, stretching my scream from molten orange to purple to black. I don't just scream for the young woman of the last three years—decades wail out of hiding. The voice that erupts doesn't belong to the girl who stayed small, who swallowed pain whole. I don't recognize her. *Who is screaming?*

She sounds pissed. She sounds worthy. She sounds alive.

* * *

For the past four years, I'd been on autopilot, dutifully following the academic steps that might bring me closer to Dad—or at least, to the life I think he wanted for me. It's still the plan. *I think*. But something is shifting. A restlessness, sharp and electric, splinters through me, threatening to pull me off course. I chose this academic and career path to feel close to him, but the question gnaws at me: *Does it? Will it ever?*

The summer after graduation, I move to Boulder, sharing a rental with Eric and his girlfriend, Kirsten. Weekdays, I work at a Montessori school. Weekends, at a flower shop. I study half-heartedly for the Medical College Admission Test, sit through the grueling exam in August, and then, to my surprise, feel something new stir in me. The first sips of life outside the health sciences are intoxicating. I fantasize about opening a flower shop. Research ethnobotany. Make a wish list of early childhood education programs around the world. All those years of pre-med—punctuated only by a rogue sociology class and dance electives—and suddenly, I'm ready to liberate my liberal arts education. As soon as I save enough money, I buy a one-way ticket to Europe. No real plan. Just a loose idea: north to south in a year. Better bring my compass.

Scotland is first. I spend three months working the organic gardens at Findhorn Foundation, a place where, in the 1970s, cabbages the size of basketballs supposedly grew because a woman talked to fairies. I never see any fairies, but darned if I try. I meditate at sunrise with Findhorn's founder, Eileen Caddy, falling into line with the simple routine of candle, cushion, breath. A welcome, if temporary, relief from the noise in my head.

I spend a brief stint at a Rudolf Steiner education center before landing here, at a Taoist retreat in Switzerland's Jungfrau mountains. I trade washing bed linens and dishes for room and board, and in exchange, the retreat director teaches me how to meditate. On my first day, he studies me for a moment, then says, "Think about nothing but your feet on the ground while you're here. That will be enough." Probably the best advice I've ever received.

I am a tall willow tree who thinks she's an air plant—roots thirsty for the ground, dangling six feet above.

On weekends, I hike mountain trails, buy blocks of goat cheese from local farms, and spend quiet evenings doodling in my journal. But don't be fooled by the serenity these scenes conjure. The outer landscape is filled with adventure, but inside, I am restless, unsatisfied, always searching. Looping thoughts poke at a pervasive sense of uncertainty. *What's my purpose? Was that a sign? What does this mean?*

My questioning is obnoxiously loud beneath the silent, assured gaze of the Alps.

I keep moving, hoping the next place will quiet the restlessness.

After ten months in Europe, I return to Colorado. I abort my travels earlier than planned because, while living at a monastery in southern France, I overhear my neighbor, a French Chinese Tibetan Buddhist monk, casually singing the John Denver tune "Take Me Home, Country Roads"—a flashing, neon arrow pointing me *home.*

Finally! A sign! I return home because the "universe" grants permission.

Lulled by familiar territory, I begin researching medical schools and exploring a growing interest in naturopathy. Dad would've loved naturopathic school and had even planted seeds to form an alternative medicine retreat center someday. Now, you can find them everywhere, but at the time his ideas were radical, perhaps even quixotic. I am inspired by his vision.

But my body has different plans. My heart starts to race. I become ravenous, eating four, five, six meals a day, but fail to dampen the sharp cry in my gut. Anxiety pokes holes in my sleep and what little I get, I awaken in pools of sweat. When I visit Mom, she's alarmed by my dramatic weight loss and insatiable appetite and takes me to the family doctor. After some Chernobyl-esque labwork involving a radioactive pill, I am diagnosed with hyperthyroidism and Grave's Disease—my thyroid is producing way too much hormone and my immune system is attacking it. Fantastic. The doc offers only one option: irradiate my thyroid and supplement the hormone synthetically.

Growing up on tofu, Celestial Seasonings tea and country air, this treatment plan feels like an foreign invasion, so I take things into my own hands. I pull *The Encyclopedia of Natural Remedies* by Louise Tenney from Mom's bookshelf, its pages soft and well-loved, the spine cracked from years of thumbing through cures. I flip to the thyroid section. Louise makes it sound easy. *Supplement with selenium and zinc! Fresh air and walks in the morning! Leafy greens. Brassicas.*

I can do this. I will fix myself.

That night, on a corner of Mom's sofa, Gray's Anatomy, Andrew Weil, Christian Northrup and Louise Hay share my lap as I research everything I can about thyroid disease. My takeaway: hyperthyroidism can be caused by the following: allergy, liver imbalance, low adrenals, stress, genes or unresolved grief.

Wait. Do I have Grave's disease because of Dad's death? Is my body attacking itself because I'm still processing? Am I still just going through the motions of grief, but not the feelings? Have I been doing this all wrong, and If I start doing it right—grieving the right way—will my thyroid heal? Will I be fixed?

I lay awake at night pleading with Dad. Sweat drips disquieted thoughts down my chest. Fits of anger surface when I drop my bowl of yoghurt on the floor or when the hammock breaks and I slam into the hardwood floor. *Where are you Dad? Why aren't you helping me?*

A few months and too much broccoli later, I see a physician known for his non-conventional approach with patients. I'm tired of being "wired and tired." He starts me on hormone therapy and suggests I remove gluten from my diet to address the autoimmune issue and candida overgrowth in my gut. Temporarily, my thyroid levels out. I stop sweating all the time, my heart rate normalizes. But this is 1998. Gluten-free diets are not a trend. This diet takes time, research and effort. My thoughts are consumed with what to, and not to, consume. Once a fun, pleasurable part of existence, now meals fill me with the dread of relapse. I trade cream cheese bagels for dry rice cakes. PB&J for buckwheat mash with peanut-butter. Black licorice for anti-fungal pills. While an honest attempt to heal my thyroid, a gluten-free diet becomes my *find-control-du-jour*. Once upon a time, I traded pliés for Clearasil. Then Clearasil for magical thinking and meditation.

And now: meditation for food hyper-vigilance and a gluten-free doughnut.

CHAPTER 10

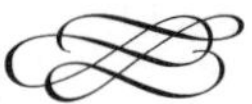

I HAVE BECOME A WANDERER.

I have little sense of what I want—except for the *universe* to tell me what I want. I no longer ask Dad to show me the way; I imagine his atoms fully dispersed, riding cosmic currents. Dad *is* the universe. I interpret events as sign posts and follow them. I find myself through others and look to them to make decisions for me. With little trust in myself, I instead trust the elusive, paternal universe. At best, this can be a great exercise in surrender and faith. But for an impressionable, fragile ego, I am left clinging to misattributions of causality in lieu of a deeper, more honest relationship with myself.

When I find myself in situations I no longer want to be in, I stubbornly persist, leaving a trail of relationship carnage behind me. *Because the universe wants me to be here. Because magic brought us together.* If I stand on my own two feet, brush off my knees and say, "I'm out of here," I am a failure of my own doing. I don't want to feel accountable for my unhappiness. I don't want to know the universe (i.e. Dad) doesn't care.

While still imperfectly managing my thyroid, I enroll in an ethnobotany course through the California Institute of Integrated Studies (CIIS) to study Ecuadorian rainforest medicines. The research director, Professor J, is dark and handsome, (thank you course catalog headshots!) and I'd be lying if that didn't factor into my decision to enroll. The possibility of meeting an interesting man heavily influences my career decisions. My lifestyle suggests I'm an independent adventurer but in truth, I look to men to define me. I have no clue who I am, much less what I want from life so I oscillate between my outdated pact with Dad to pursue medicine and tethering myself to a boy, letting his lift sculpt the outline of mine.

The CIIS course is a perfect blend of both, so in early spring I fly to Ecuador to study tropical rainforest plants and meet my new ethnobotanist husband. It's clear within minutes of meeting Professor J that he's unavailable and uninterested so I redirect my thoughts to magical thinking and the green spirits of the jungle. *Maybe when I'm two days down the Amazon River and away from civilization, plants will finally talk to me.* The class convenes briefly in Quito and then a large bus escorts us from clouds to rainforest floor—over 8000 foot elevation drop—arriving at a concrete hostel after dark for a short night's sleep.

Just past midnight, I vomit my way to the bathroom and fall asleep on the cool floor hugging the toilet, only to be awakened by pounding on my locked door at 6am. Delirious, emptied, but better, I splash water on my face and answer the door—it's time to go. I grab my backpack and make a note-to-self: no more roadside chicken.

We travel another few hours on the winding, asphalt Amazon, descending into its vibrant, more fluid realm. I keep my gaze fixed out the window, hues of gray dotted with the vibrant reds and blues of Ecuadorian textiles eventually yield to a wall of green.

After another eight hours—wheels giving way to motorized canoe—we finally arrive. Shamans Don Elijio, Don Cesario and their families greet us barefoot, smiles mirroring the wide, ochre shoreline they stand upon. When the two elders and Professor J embrace, it's clear their long-standing and mutually beneficial transaction has also nurtured a deep friendship. We unload gear and are ushered to a large, open palapa where cassava, plantain and beans restore our weary bodies. This is my first real meal since the roadside *campylobacter*. I feel light-headed and disoriented but the two giggly children flanking my side invite my cells to land. I am nurtured as much by the meal as their rooted, unquestioning bodies.

Following dinner, we are instructed to find sleeping spots. I grab my tarp and mosquito net, scanning the sprawling rainforest as the last of the light dissolves into shadow.

"You can set up anywhere," the elders say, "just not over there."

They gesture toward the far end of the property. I follow their hands but see only darkness, jungle folding into itself. I skirt just south of the forbidden area and, in the dimming light, make out the silhouette of a round structure with a large, thatched roof in the distance. A narrow path, tangled on both sides by heavy, twisted vines, beckons toward the entrance.

Exhausted from food poisoning and two days of travel, I drop my tarp on a cleared patch near the path and collapse into sleep.

I dream of fire. The group is gathered around a pyre of skeletons, our voices low at first, a quiet chant rising as the flames grow. We stand, we dance, circling the blaze, and as the bones catch fire, flesh returns. Muscle, sinew, and skin knit together with each note. The more we sing and dance, the more the skeletons disappear—until fully formed women step from the flames, whole, reborn.

At dawn, murmured voices pull me from sleep. I blink up at the sky, liminal chanting still thrumming in my brain. A few feet away, Don Cesario and Professor J nod in greeting before continuing their conversation, their words lost on me—*high school French be damned*. I fumble for my flip-flops, unsure of what to do, and slip away. Later, over breakfast, the director chuckles as he approaches. "Kim, you're sleeping in the middle of a sacred ayahuasca garden."

Ayahuasca, or yagé, is a vine that grows predominantly in South America and is used for spiritual ceremony among indigenous tribes. Don Cesario and Don Elijio have both "journeyed" with yagé two hundred times in about as many days—part of their initiation as shamans. In Quechua, *aya* means "spirit, soul" or "corpse", and *huaska* means "rope" and "woody vine." People across the globe partake in these ceremonies, some traveling to South American rainforests, others drinking the concoction in the nave of their local Christian church. Many extoll the revelatory powers of the medicine—finding their purpose, downloading secrets of the universe, healing trauma or talking with the deceased.

Only academically familiar with ayahuasca, I am intrigued to learn the medicine is nearby. But as I sit at a long table over breakfast, listening more than talking, it becomes clear the vine's presence is not an accident. It is actually the *raison d'être* for the entire ethnobotanical journey. We're not here to study a diversity of Ecuadorian rainforest plants. We're here to study one—yagé.

After the vine is boiled down to a potent tea, the group prepares for the journey. Women on their menstrual cycles are forbidden to participate so I'm eliminated from the ceremonies. I'm relieved. Other than a few memorable trips with ecstasy and psilocybin in college, my body and drugs aren't a friendly match. I'm the girl who stares blankly at a wall after smoking a little weed. Or worse, passes out. No matter, I'm sleeping in the ayahuasca patch. Oddly, I'm not banished from the sacred garden so I reason the vines will speak through my dreams instead.

After a day of fasting, the participants are ready. What I don't realize about my vine garden accommodation is that it is also in earshot of the ceremonial palapa. Before yagé takes effect, it barrels through one's GI tract like a freight train. My romantic notion of sleeping with the sounds of the rainforest end here. Instead of rhythmic chirping and the gentle rustling of palms, my lullabies are violent retching and bowel explosions. And once the vine's shape-shifting hallucinations take effect, I am lulled to sleep by *Homo sapiens* yowling with phantom fur.

To this day, I am unsure how I overlooked the central purpose of the trip. Or did the course catalog cloak it in more generic, ethnobotanical terms so as to avoid scrutiny? I don't know. But each day, while the rest of the group recovers in hammocks before the next ceremony, I put on my rubber wellies and hike through the forest. My senses push off loneliness by consuming the thick, wet persistence of photosynthesis and survival.

Naively, I don't wear socks with my boots. By the end of the trek, my heels are raw, the skin peeled away to reveal large oozing sores. Each evening, I soak my open wounds in the muddy riverbank, convinced the cool water will soothe. A few days later, a fever grips me in its teeth. My body burns, then shivers, drenching my sleeping pad in a sweat as I drift in and out of a fitful sleep.

I'm not the only one. Two others fall ill—later diagnosed with Hepatitis C. The elders agree it's time to ship out. We make our way to Quito, dosing ourselves with trusted pharmaceuticals, but the altitude at 9,000 feet turns every breath into a battle. Desperate for relief, we flee to the coast—a short flight, and a cab ride later, we check into a remote hostería by the sea, hoping the waves will wash our sickness away.

Why did I have to come all this way, only to feel miserable? I've had no revelations. Even the ayahuasca remained silent. My body is weak, sustained on fried plantains and rice. I don't know what foreign bacteria is vacationing in my blood, but I struggle to keep anything down. I fade in and out of sleep, fever dreams threading through me:

I am swimming. Or maybe I'm sinking? I hover, weightless, near the ocean floor. A faint light reaches from above and a dolphin swims through the pale-blue cylinder.

And in the anything-goes manner of dreams…

The dolphin introduces himself to me. "My name is Ambato. Follow me."

The next day, feeling a bit better than terrible, I'm sitting at the hostel's outdoor patio when a mob of tan, sun-bleached men descends on a nearby table. Tiny sensors in my cochlea snap to attention, searching for a lifeline, but all I catch are "sick waves" and "off-shore winds." A few men have large video cameras at their sides, wet longboards strewn around them. With magical thinking as my warmest bedfellow, I quickly spin a narrative where this entourage holds the meaning I came here to find. *Maybe a new love—or better, my soulmate—is among them. Maybe the camera crew needs an assistant, and I'll fall into an exciting new career in film.* The heat, my empty stomach and even emptier heart make me delirious for serendipity.

Impulsively, I walk over to a younger-looking man with kind eyes and introduce myself. His sandy blonde curls are tied into a messy ponytail, his jaw is wide and strong and the Australian accent that falls from it makes my heart flutter. He is shy, but so am I. We volley a few tentative questions"—Hey, who are you?" What are you doing here?"—before I privately cast myself in the final act of their film,

Secret Spot, a longboard surf documentary about undiscovered Ecuadorian waves. The professional surfers are on their last leg up the coast, catching a few fun rides today before heading home.

At last, with a *choose-my-own-adventure* ending in reach, I head to the beach that afternoon to watch my fantasy soulmate surf.

His name is Beau. Of course it is.

While walking back to my room, the dream resurfaces. *The dolphin's name was "Ambato." I'm sure of it. But am I? Maybe I remembered it wrong. Maybe it was Beau. Maybe it was abbreviated? Maybe he said, "My name is Ambato, but you can call me Beau?"*

That sounds right. It must be right.

The more I think about it, the more I convince myself THIS IS WHY I CAME TO ECUADOR! THIS IS WHY I GOT SICK! THIS JOURNEY WAS LEADING ME HERE, TO MEET BEAU.

Late that afternoon, after Beau rides a few last waves, we sip tea on the beach, exchange a friendly kiss, contact info, and goodbyes.

When I return to the States, a message is waiting. "Hey, one of my board sponsors is in Japan. I'm headed there in a month. Come meet me."

And I do. We spend a few months in Japan, then another year living together in Australia. Beau's Japanese friends loosely translate my name—*KinBaRi*—to mean *Golden Wings Return Home*. I oblige. The eastern hemisphere becomes my new home.

* * *

But spring comes, as it does, and I receive an acceptance letter for the Naturopathic College of Natural Medicine (NCNM) in Oregon. I abruptly end my twelve month relationship with Beau and exit the eastern hemisphere. Occasional thyroid storms, an unhappy gut riddled with South American critters, and aimless apathy contribute to my decision. Beau's gentle way never deserved my fickle heart.

I move to Portland and live alone in a small apartment. I like the city—or at least, the *idea* of it. I meet new friends and envy their artistic careers, their effortless way of moving through the world, untethered to their bodies.

I am anything but untethered. My awareness is locked in a relentless orbit around my own flesh—uncomfortable sensations, constant body scanning, intrusive thoughts, hyper-vigilance. Despite three years of expanded horizons, I am still a young woman with only one lens in her camera bag: *wellness.*

Occasionally, during restless, hyperthyroid nights, I have access to a wider angle. Underneath the noise, I long to be someone else, to see the world through a different lens. I feel a creative whim, however outdated, that is still dancing on stage or building imaginary worlds with my childhood friend Jenny. The summer before NCNM begins I scour local Craigslist ads and land a two month gig at North Shore Productions, a small, documentary film company. *Perfect. I'm ready for my new life in Hollywood.*

My first day at work, I receive a giant cardboard box filled with DVDs, VHS and Beta-Cam tapes. A local organization, Dougy Center, hired North Shore to create their 25th anniversary video and I am to watch and log their historical content. *Sure! What's the Dougy Center? No clue, no matter!* I'm relieved to have an interim new focus. I open my notebook, grab a VHS tape on top of the pile, and queue it up.

Within the first ten minutes, I learn that the Dougy Center provides support for children, teens, young adults, and their families grieving the death of a loved one. *Gulp.* I have hundreds upon hundreds of hours of logging ahead of me. Lectures by grief specialists and founders. Bereavement groups with children. Tours around the facility. Teens, young adults and parents talking about their experiences of suicide, murder, cancer and sudden accidents.

One of the tapes is titled *Beverly Chappell, 1989*. Beverly, founder and former nurse, envisioned a place where children, teens, and their parents coping with death could share their experiences in a safe, compassionate community. In this particular footage she speaks to educators about signs of unhealthy or unresolved grief. I listen and take notes.

But then I stop. Rewind. Play the segment again.

I stare at the screen, synapses in a sudden scramble. The pen slips from my fingers and I begin sweating.

Beverly explains different grief responses to the educators.

"Some children act out in the classroom after a death. Others retreat, become quiet. In both cases, their behavior shifts—a sign they are *feeling* something. Sure, they'll need guidance, but their cry for help is heard."

She goes on.

"But then, there are the ones that go unnoticed. They become perfectionists. They keep to their plans. All we see are successful, well-adjusted kids. They graduate at the top of their class, go off to college or start careers."

And then—surely breaking the fourth wall—she looks into my eyes.

"Usually five to ten years or so following the death, when that child or adolescent is now a young adult, we start to see problems. And in many cases, these problems are physical. The body breaks down under the stress of unresolved grief."

There's that paring of words again: unresolved grief. *The body breaks down under the stress of unresolved grief.*

The next day I sign up for a six day volunteer training at the Dougy Center.

I end up volunteering on and off for over six years. One spring, not too long after my initial training, I help develop a bereavement theater troupe for young adults. Talk circles don't often feel like enough, especially as kids mature. Teens and young adults don't just want to *talk* about grief—they want *do* something with it. They want to act out, create, make it real in a way words alone can't.

My friend Lauren brings her experience from a similar troupe in Eugene, Oregon and I bring empathy and enthusiasm. For four months, a remarkable, tortured and sensitive group of young adults craft a stage performance, calling themselves the *Scarlett Ds*—D for death, of course.

During my favorite skit, the entire troupe lines up on stage, backs facing the audience. They introduce their grief stories with simple commands. "Turn around if your mom died." "Turn around if your dad died." Sometimes just one Scarlet D turns around. Sometimes a handful.

Then, more details. "Turn around if it was a suicide." "Turn around if you got to say goodbye." The audience grows silent. Feet stop shuffling. Eyes fix on the performers' heart-wrenching realities.

Then, the final command.

"Turn around if you'd give up everything you've learned since your person died, in order to have them back."

Not a single one of the Scarlett Ds turns around.

During rehearsals, we worked with this question a lot. Some days they wanted to erase all the lessons, just to be back in their daddy's arms. But most days, they were in consensus. "Navigating grief has made me a better person." "Now I know how to connect with others in pain." "I understand now that it's okay to not be okay."

These conclusions are not provoked. The Scarlet Ds like the versions of themselves that have been dragged into the slaughter house, necks exposed to the sharp and unforgiving blade of loss. They cherish new bonds and celebrate a resiliency they never knew they had.

The audience is stunned. During the Q&A, a few people are even threatened. One middle-aged woman raises her hand and in an accusatory tone asks, "How can you choose your own growth over the life of another?"

The Scarlett Ds reply with the maturity of a thousand sages, "It doesn't have to be so black and white. Of course, we want our loved ones back. But we don't get to choose what happens to us, we can only choose how it shapes us. And we like who we've become."

CHAPTER 11

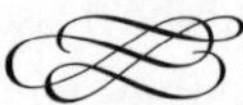

When I begin my medical training at National College of Naturopathic Medicine (NCNM), I yearn for a different path but with no clear direction, medicine is my default. During the first week, I sit in the back of *Intro to Human Physiology* and draw pencil sketches of classmates, not because I'm an illustrator, but because I'm trying to be someone else. I'm pretending to be one of the cool, free-spirited artists who sell their work at Portland's Last Thursday art events. I want to drop out, return to my summer gig at North Shore Productions and learn how to edit or join their film crew.

At lunch, I eavesdrop on classmates discussing herbs, nutrition, and yoga—their voices reverent, their certainty unwavering. I judge them for their dogma, then judge myself for the same. My wellness-dominated neuroses are perfectly at home at NCNM.

But what about the rest of me?

A week later, a little under a month into my graduate training, two commercial airlines fly into the World Trade Center. I see the sudden national uncertainty as a sign, always a sign, to dive into my own. I drop out.

Aside from a bimonthly volunteering commitment at the Dougy Center, I am lost and craving structure. Through a connection at a local gym, I land a receptionist job at Downstream, a post-production film company. I don't experience the craft firsthand, but I enjoy the clients and the easygoing conversations at the front desk.

No one talks about self-improvement. No one mentions gluten. It's refreshing.

Most of Downstream's work is commercial—animation spots for Nickelodeon, infomercials for vacuum cleaners and freight services. No Academy Award contenders, not even inspiring indie shorts. The directors sometimes mock their own projects—"Another Saturday morning ad for kids jacked on Cocoa Krispies." But I envy them.

There's something about the script-to-final-cut collaboration that reminds me of ballet—the long, disciplined arc of choreography, training, rehearsing, and performance. The work itself may be uninspiring, but a meaningless sense of purpose, one that smells nothing of herbal remedies and incense, is strangely enlivening.

Occasionally, during quiet evenings at home I play with iMovie on my laptop. I make insanely stupid videos of my friend's dog, walks in the park, derivative observations from a bus stop bench. I enroll in a few classes at the NW Film Center. I take a writing course at The Attic. But instead of feeling inspired, I feel disoriented. Fraudulent. Like I'm playing a part in a film I didn't make—because I'm not a real filmmaker.

I'm also afraid. After a deluge of medical emergencies and relentless physical discomforts, my body has become omnipresent alarm. Some specialists refer to this as "Medical PTSD." I am a walking, ticking, time bomb. Blinding menstrual cramps that leave me face-planted on the floor or blacked-out on airline passengers' laps. Sudden, violent illness strikes without warning. My gut is a battlefield. My thyroid, a volatile storm. Food hyper-vigilance balloons into body hyper-vigilance. I constantly scan for sensations that may signify impending danger. Once an unsafe world, the walls close in—now my body feels unsafe.

Determined to get to the root of my health problems, I visit a highly recommended physician in Arizona, where Mom now resides with a former Wooster College alum. A few times a year, I fly down and spend days at the clinic, hooked up to IV drips of acetaminophen and mercury detox formulas.

The IV clinic feels more like a waiting room for the half-dead. Reclining chairs line the entire circumference of the room, filled with pale, sunken-eyed patients—two or three at a time, including me. The space is oddly pedestrian, like the lounge of a low-budget convalescent home—muted beige walls, stiff vinyl recliners, a stack of outdated magazines no one picks up. A tired artificial plant droops in the corner, as if it, too, has been here too long. I bring a book but mostly, steal glances at the others, searching their faces for some sign of improvement. *Is this working for any of us? Isn't this supposed to make us feel better?*

The doctor determines—through a highly suspicious "machine"—that I'm allergic to nearly every food, chemical, and molecule on God's green earth. The machine itself looks like something pulled from the back of a junk drawer, about the size of a Webster's Dictionary, with an analog feel that makes it seem both outdated and oddly mystical. I extend my finger, and he presses it against a cold metal pad while a tiny vial containing the "allergen" rests on the other side. No needles, no blood, just this strange, unspoken alchemy of skin, metal, and glass.

The verdict? I need homeopathic vials for each of my offenders—seven drops per vial, three times a day, for upwards of 30 different substances.

This isn't sustainable. I spiral into a black-hole of obsessive, compulsive thinking: *Will this oil paint trigger my thyroid? But I want to be an artist! Will this dank classroom make my brain foggy? But I want to learn! Does this soy sauce have gluten? But I want to go out with friends! Did I get parasites overseas? But I love traveling! If I drink this glass of wine will I feel terrible tomorrow? But I want to have fun! Why isn't my brain working today? Who cares!*

I become a two-headed monster, and my shoulder-mates do not get along. Kim 1 wants to celebrate chaos, play, vulnerability, and uncertainty. Kim 2 needs control to survive. Their uproar is deafening.

Once a month, around the raging chaos of hormones, I begin purging—confusing emptiness with peace.

I check out books from the library and try to understand the behavior. But it's 2002. Purging Disorder isn't an official diagnosis yet and everything I read points to bulimia and anorexia but I don't relate. I don't binge and I'm not trying to influence my body shape or weight.

Blaming eating disorders on body image issues feels one-dimensional. Women have complex, powerfully emotional lives and we carry centuries of generational trauma in our bodies. Our DNA is not foreign to invasion, perpetration, and silencing. The world is uncertain and through a perfect storm of circumstances, I now distrust my body's ability to handle it. When I purge, I'm saying no to the world when my body can't.

I purge to be quiet. I purge to be still. I purge to be safe. I purge to be at peace. And yet.

I feel violent helplessness in the act and then soft connection afterwards. Looking in the mirror, eyes bloodshot and watering, I dialog with this undone version of myself. *Who am I? What do I want?* Below the questioning, I am just seconds, a-fraction-of-a-second, away from the answer. *Like remembering a sequence of notes from a dream and if I could just hold on a bit longer, I'd recall the entire melody.*

I feel reckless but honest. Out-of-control but vibrating with newness and possibility. *I hear the notes! I hear you at last!* When emptied, I feel like *me*—innocent, intact, untouched by anything or anyone else's influence. No one telling me how to act, what to believe, how to heal, and most of all, who to be.

For a spell, control and chaos co-exist and the two-headed monster becomes one.

But the safety is only temporary. A sinking feeling always returns. A complete and total loss of control. And grief. So much grief. Unresolved.

I experiment with purging for two years. Sometimes once every few months. Other times, every week. But it never becomes a habit, never escalates, never takes on a life of its own the way I fear it might. But it never fully disappears either. It comes and goes, an unruly guest that arrives unannounced, stays just long enough to take up space, then vanishes—only to return again. Always within the same cycle: control, loss of control, guilt, repentance.

It never helps, not really. Except in those fleeting moments right afterward—the eerie, weightless calm, the strange hum of *me, only me*. As if I've emptied out all the noise, the expectations, the voices that aren't mine. For a brief window, I exist in pure quiet, resting in the emptiness of myself. But it fades and when it does, I'm left in the same body, with the same unanswered ache.

The cycle doesn't evolve. It doesn't deepen, doesn't spiral, doesn't demand more from me. It simply repeats itself, frozen in time. And then, one day, without ceremony—no epiphany, no reckoning—only a deliberate, willful decision, it disappears completely.

But the two-headed monster is always near, subdued by distraction or afire with strife. My body submits, longing to be their altar of unification.

JULY 13, 2003

Dear Charlie,

Almost everyone owns a home computer now. Sometimes I stay up late, laptop my divination tool. The curser blinks in the empty search bar mocking my own vacancy. I type "Who am I" but Google thinks Christian rock YouTube videos are my answer.

Mom and I spoke earlier on the phone and your name came up. Again. Over the years, she's told the story a handful of times—always the same details, always the same wistful tone. A chance encounter, a fleeting connection, a longing to know herself in a new way. It's become something of a family joke—her Free Love phase, condensed to a single evening.

And now, I'm part of the joke too. We all laugh about it, the absurdity of it, the microscopic chance that you're actually my dad. No one ever takes it seriously, not for a second. No even me. But still, when I hear your name—Charlie—it lingers like a forgotten tune.

So with digital tea-leaves at my fingertips and a half-hearted sense of amusement, I search again. Charlie Bower. Charlie Brewer. Charlie Wisconsin Public Access Television. Charlie musician.

German actor born in 1935 aside, the results offer nothing remotely resembling the "you" Mom describes. I let it go.

CHAPTER 12

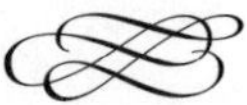

I KEEP SIGNING up for classes at NW Film Center and The Attic—hoping something will take. Amidst my physical challenges, these courses inspire me. Improv and Meisner stretch me. A community psychology course at Portland State, a hospice training with Roshi Joan Halifax, and bereavement groups at the Dougy Center pull me toward meaning. Meanwhile, for two whole years, I sample careers like hors d'oeuvres at a party. I answer phones at Downstream, fold blouses at a friend's boutique, sign with a modeling agency, and step into small film roles and commercials. I am everywhere and nowhere, skimming the surface of possibility, waiting for something to stick.

My outer life feels big and unrestricted. The inner landscape, not so much, but the horizon is widening.

One of Dad's favorite tee's used to read, *Life is mysterious, don't take it so serious.* As a teen, the dismembered adverb drove me insane—a grammar worm eating itself through my brain demanding I sharpie a fat "LY" at the end of "serious." I missed the point—the great mystery pinched between a rule and a rule-follower.

Now, I'm letting that mystery breathe. The reclaimed oxygen ignites a creative fire within.

My new manifesto proclaims: Create. Stop thinking so hard.

Fail. Make a fool out of yourself. Embrace meaninglessness. Do what feels good. Stop hiding. Risk being lost, embarrassed, nervous, judged, misinterpreted, and unloved.

And most importantly, don't turn the manifesto into a new psycho-spiritual goal.

But the fire is too hot. Excitement crackles through me, indistinguishable from stress, my body unable to tell the difference. My nervous system doesn't parse joy from danger; it only knows arousal, acceleration, the relentless churn of *too much.* I forget to contain the flames. Soon my thyroid shows signs of alarming imbalance again. My resting heart rate elevates to 125. I can't stand upright without feeling dizzy. I sweat and shake constantly. I develop insomnia. In three months, I drop from a healthy 135 to 115. I see a cardiologist. An endocrinologist. I revisit the drip-of-death in Arizona and deteriorate after each treatment. "That's good," the doctor says, "your body is ridding itself of toxins!" I start back up on my giant clutch of homeopathic vials. I juice. I do yin yoga. I start meditating again. I buy expensive supplements. And I purge when overwhelmed, sitting *sukhasana* at my porcelain altar, resting at ground zero.

And just like that, I lose enthusiasm for the mystery. I need safety, comfort and familiarity. I need everything to slow…way… down.

I am a child sitting under the dinner table. Above my laminate horizon are too many voices, too many lights, too much static. In my dark linen enclosure, I disappear into every bad carpet in every bad restaurant in Wisconsin. The smells, patterns, and erratic animation of conversing shoes dampen my overwhelm. I prefer it down here—quiet, safe, away from the human realm. When the world is too much, darkness and a dank carpet are good friends.

But now I'm an adult and it's not appropriate to sit under the table at Dragon Gate and read discarded fortunes. I begin to wonder if I've discarded my own.

I need a path. I need something structured, steady—something known. I need a way to move forward without needing to constantly ask where I'm going.

Panting, panicked and ten feet above my body, I see an MD/ND/DCOM—west and east harmonized in the mind of one, talented physician—a few blocks from my apartment. Within a few miraculous months on corticosteroids, my heart rate slows. I am no longer dizzy standing at the grocery check-out. I stop sprinting through time toward an early death. I return to my normal weight. My thoughts slow, unravel, soften. I am still. I am here.

And medicine is here too. Not as revelation, not as redemption, but as a path I understand. A way to be useful. A way to escape the weight of my own uncertainty.

So in September 2003, I walk through the front doors of NCNM (again) and recommit to a career in medicine. *Yes, this will be good. This will be me.*

* * *

During my first year back at NCNM (now called NUNM), I meet Dave on a commercial photoshoot. Straddling school with occasional modeling jobs somewhat pacifies my creative inclinations. On this gig, I'm booked as a "yogini" for a Nike Mother's Day video. Dave, a creative director, is on a neighboring set. Face caked with enough foundation to flatten me into two dimensions, I wait for my cue to fold in half. I'm a pretend yogi, but I know the poses. Sorta.

During a three-hour wait, I curl up in a vacant chair and open my book. Next to me, a man with messy, salt-and-pepper hair and a ~~5:00~~ 5 *day* shadow, works a Nike wristwatch design on his open laptop. We exist in easy, parallel silence. I read. I nap. His mouse glides across the trackpad, a quiet metronome between us. When I wake up, he asks about my book. I'm only mildly invested in the novel, but the conversation it sparks—the exchange of our favorites—pulls me in. Dave just finished reading the horror novel *Perfume*. Whereas I just finished reading *The Spell of the Sensuous: Perception and Language in a More-Than-Human World*. Eventually we exchange email addresses to elaborate on our lists. I don't think much of it until a week later I receive his email:

Subject: (no subject)
Perfume
Dandelion Wine
The Terror
(503.704.8938)

quid pro quo

I happen to be in a relationship with another man. We live together but in the last few months have drifted apart. I don't end things with him—a decision too emancipated for this version of Kim—but when Dave's "quid pro quo" develops into one-email-a-week, one-a-day, then emails all-day-long, any last thread of emotional connection with the other man dissolves. He exits within 24 hours of discovering months of email exchanges with Dave. Moving out his box of designer shoes is heavier than the break-up.

Though we live only seven miles apart, Dave and I continue our written correspondence. These aren't your typical "Hey, how are you" emails. Writing Dave is like attending a workshop with Raymond Carver—keep it simple, pay attention to the little things, focus on the ordinary over the extraordinary.

I develop a Pavlovian heart flutter every time my email chimes. Between classes I run to NUNM'S computer lab, an addict craving her next hit. Dave's raw, poetic honesty solicits the same from me, and I become grounded in an emotional truth I haven't felt for years, maybe ever. Always a direct line into my heart, an alien with two bald heads could woo me with good prose. Luckily, Dave is from planet Earth and has enough hair on his *one* head for five men.

And then there's this: Dave. Dad's name. And his middle name: Charles. *Of course it is.*

He's also 43 when we meet—Dad's recurrent, quiet signal from beyond.

A part of me feels oddly comforted by these details, as if Dad is still nearby, nudging me toward something, toward him. Toward whatever comes next.

During our four-months of monogamous pen-pal-ing, I learn Dave and his ex (married young, divorced young) share custody of their eleven year-old daughter Syd. "She's different," he writes and doesn't expand.

And later, in another email: "Syd's experience of the world is unlike mine or yours."

With time and trust, he shares more: her harrowing entry into this world; the endless seizures; his abandonment of religion because it sure doesn't feel like "God's way" and the comfort he felt when his brother tells him, simply "This is shit"; the doctor's prognosis, "She won't ever walk or eat unassisted"; and their early morning, frame-assisted strolls through an empty mall because he insists she *will* walk someday. His love for her is wide and deep.

On Saturdays Dave and Syd like to wander Portland's popular Knob Hill neighborhood. I live a few blocks away, so I meet them at a sidewalk table-for-two at Torrefazzione Coffee House. I haven't encountered much, if any, disability in my life and am ashamed of my naiveté. As I approach, I want to be open and casual but I feel like anything but.

I see Dave's disheveled mane first. His Chuck Taylors. His, I don't-give-a-fuck attitude pulls me in like good gravity—steady, undeniable. Across the table, a blond head hunches over, carefully scooping up a child-size vanilla ice cream. Both our spinning slows in his orbit—my nervous system, always seeking ground, and Syd's tangled synapses, always firing, finding equilibrium in his pull.

I crouch by the table as Syd looks over and asks, "What time it is?" The phrasing catches me off guard, but I glance at my watch and answer. Five minutes later, she asks again. And again.

Her insistence is code for something else. For what, we will never know, but Syd's conversations are never random. Maybe she's reaching into a memory. Maybe she's making a connection. I feel clumsy in our exchanges, like I'm learning a new language. And self-conscious. Forever trying to fit in, and now, in the company of Dave and Syd, I will never. We will never. Grocery store clerks, passersby, waiters—all make that painfully clear. Under their bewildered stares, I am a teenager again with cover-up caked pimples afraid of everything I can't hide.

Dave has no June Cleaver expectations. Parenting a child with intellectual disability, he's learned that life is messy, outcomes unpredictable, often unwanted. Granted, Jack Daniels is his current therapist, but his surrendered comfort with the oft darkness of reality draws me in.

I am a sun-deprived plant bending toward the light, but in reverse.

The following Saturday, Dave offers to help change the bolt lock on my door. While he works, Syd and I listen to Imogen Heap on repeat. She sings along, eyes squinting, face lifted toward a certain, celestial partner.

Mid-doorknob assembly and a quiet pause between tracks, I share, “I love having you and Syd in my home.”

Dave’s eyes redden and liquify, heart leaping out through salty waters.

The next morning he texts, *I was so flustered after you said that, I accidentally installed the bolt lock on the wrong side of your door.*

Oh, the ache. All three of us, longing to belong.

At times, Syd frightens me. Not in any rational, nameable way. It’s the absence of a map, the way I can’t find my usual handholds for connection. I ask her a question, and she repeats it back to me—a perfect echo, the words intact but hollow, as if their meaning has slipped through some unseen crack before reaching her. Or me. I don’t know how to get to her, and the absence of that knowing panics me.

And then there are the things I do know—the things I feel in my body before my brain can rationalize. Her sudden vocal outbursts that spike my nervous system, the way my muscles clench at the sound, the primitive urge to run. The smell of urine in her room, the stacks of damp sheets, the way my stomach tightens when I hear Dave peeling them off her bed again. The daily reminders that Syd isn’t fixed, will never be, and I’m not ready to meet that in myself.

I spent my whole life bracing against what can’t be controlled. My body has been trying to teach me this lesson for years but I’ve treated it like a project—something that, with just the right thing, could be corrected. Syd’s body holds another kind of lesson, one I am even less prepared to receive. She’s unshaped by expectation. She moves at her own pace, follows her own script, exists beyond all the usual markers of progress.

And Dave doesn’t encourage an opening. Eleven years of single-parenting in his bones, he’s also learned to not depend on anyone—fathering a daughter who talks funny, engages differently, will never live independently. He doesn’t ask me to help, doesn’t expect me to love her, never requests I step in and step up.

So, I do as I’ve done before. For better and/or worse. I compartmentalize. While my love for Dave deepens, I wade in the kiddy pool with Syd. I mostly engage through attempts to fix her. Gluten-free diets! Music Therapy! Bodywork! DNA sequencing! Fish oil! I've been down these paths before. I research, I ask professors at school for advice, I present treatments to Dave, we try things, I grumble about Syd's mom not following *the new plan* (and blame her when it doesn't work), and then try something new. I never lose hope because that's not an option.

But what am I really hoping for?

I learn to connect, not with Syd, but with the possibility of Syd. Not with her unique expression in this world, but wrongly, with the one I want—the one I refuse to accept for myself. The one who isn't broken. The one who simply is.

CHAPTER 13

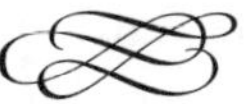

Dave and I are sound asleep. And then, we are not.

Startled awake by cellular alarm bells, I sit up, disoriented. Something isn't right. My body knows before I do. I clutch the bed, my voice unfamiliar as I ask Dave to get me some water.

By the time he returns, I am gone.

Unconscious, sprawled in a body that has betrayed me—urine, excrement, the remnants of control abandoned. A black hole squeezes me into singularity. Somewhere in the distance, Dave calls 911.

I come to as an EMT carries me down the stairs, strapped to the rigid certainty of a gurney. A searing pain floods my lower abdomen, recedes, then floods again. I am a tide, rolling in and out of consciousness, pulled into an undertow I cannot fight.

I hear voices on the other side of a thick, rubber wall, "Are you diabetic?" "Could you be pregnant?" "Do you have epilepsy?" My voice replies from a distant shore. "No, no. No." And then another flame burns through me. I disappear into reassuring black.

* * *

Seven days earlier, I sit with Dr. Werner Heim, a world-renowned Chinese medicine scholar and founding professor of NUNM's Classical Chinese Medicine program (CCM), at his clinic east of Portland. When he's not reading academic papers or doing research, he has a thriving practice treating chronic, difficult and recalcitrant diseases with Chinese herbs. As an enthusiastic transfer into the school's new CCM curriculum, I feel a strong affinity for Eastern medicine, its elegant understanding of science and symbolism, and Dr. Heim's integration of the two. I also enjoy my visits to his home clinic—an idyllic, off-grid womb of nature and family. He frequently treats students at NUNM—an opportunity to witness "the master in action"—to help our sleep-deprived brains function optimally during the rigors of academia. I see him in my never-ending quest for a thyroid fix, but more, I recognize Dr. Heim as a father figure. I am calmed and hopeful in his wise, healing presence.

While my right hand rests on his desk, Dr. Heim runs his usual gamut of tests. In Chinese medicine, a patient's pulse and tongue are primary diagnostic tools. Dr. Heim instead uses a clunky-looking device from Germany that I'd sooner see in an auto body shop than health clinic. It's eerily similar to the Arizona doc's machine but I suppress suspicions. Students and faculty alike extol Dr. Heim's excellence so we trust, maybe even deify him.

He places a sensor on my index finger, then taps a number of keys. Testing, assessing, scribbling notes. Testing, assessing, more scribbles. No words are exchanged. I hand over a weightless faith and relax in the hearth of familiar, fatherly care.

"Hm." He says.

"Hm?" I reply.

"Your kidneys are cold. The yang qi is very deficient, almost non-existent."

In Chinese medicine, kidneys represent the ancestral energy we inherit in the form of talents, life purpose and opportunities. Yang is the expansive, active form of this energy and is connected to the masculine—the father. YANG was also Dad's license plate.

Dr. Heim looks at me and says, "It's as if your ancestral father line is missing or empty."

I reply matter of factly. "Well, my dad died when I was 18."

He's not satisfied with my answer. "There's something more," he says. "The degree of "cold" in your yang kidney channel feels bigger than the loss of your father." He makes a note to add an herb to my formula that will rouse the yang deficiency.

The herb is called Fu Zi, or Aconite. Also known as *Monks-hood*, these prayerful, purple hermits belie their innocence—ingesting just two milligrams is fatal. Chinese herbalists have been using this plant for centuries for its ability to revive and warm severely deficient or contracted symptoms. Herbs are classified with specific properties—hot, cold, pungent, bitter, sour, or sweet. Aconite is one of the hottest plants used in Chinese Medicine. Not hot to touch, of course. Hot because, when administered, it's like jumpstarting a dead battery. Many practitioners avoid using it, but Dr. Heim has successfully healed patients, including his own cardiac tumor, using this powerful herb.

So when Dr. Heim suggests adding Aconite to my formula, I oblige. The potential to heal nagging autoimmunity *and* my "empty or missing ancestral father line" is too compelling to ignore. Cautious but obliging, I start taking the brown, acrid smelling powder.

Within a day, the herb fulfills her prophesy. My skin becomes hot. My head, even hotter. Exhaling, I feel like an open-flame pizza oven. During a diagnosis exercise in my Herbs II class, a friend reports, "Kim, your tongue is black."

I stop taking the formula but Dr. Heim suggests a lower dose. *Aconite is doing its job. I just need less voltage*. I see myself at the end of a long journey—little purple-hooded monks ushering me home. With broken circuit repaired, grief's long blackout will finally lift, light returning to the very marrow of me.

For six nights straight, I dream of dying. A shark tears into me. Lightning splits me in two. A tsunami drags me under, and I don't resurface. A chemical bomb detonates, and I dissolve into a million burning pieces. In thirty years, I can count my nightmares on one hand. Now, my brain has subscribed to terror, a nightly horror reel I can't cancel.

Meanwhile, in waking life, my body keeps the theme. A fever

climbs. My first-ever bladder infection rages. Over the phone, my doctor prescribes Cipro—just in case things spiral further.

I feel hot, sluggish, disoriented. Dave thinks it's the flu. He picks up my prescription, and at 5 p.m., I take my first dose.

In six hours, the EMTs will arrive.

I spend the night in the ER, slipping in and out of consciousness. At 2 a.m., Dave calls Mom—their first-ever conversation—and reassures her, "We're in the ER, but Kim is going to be okay."

I cling to his words, clawing my way back from nothingness, then slipping under again. When I finally stabilize, a kind nurse layers one, two, then three warm, weighted blankets over me. My muscles shiver, throwing off adrenaline.

Calmed at last, I return to what I know: It's early morning. Spring 2006. I am a student. A girlfriend. A daughter. I survived.

But here's what I don't know: Why it happened. Why the flag of uncertainty claims my body as its nation. The attending physician conjectures. Possible seizure? Allergy to Cipro? Renal colic? Aconite isn't considered; in Western medicine, these mischievous purple monk plants are ignored. The ER doctor can only confidently report the reaction, not the cause. "Kimberly Warner experienced a strong vasovagal response."

***Cause*: Unknown.**

***Reaction*: Unconsciousness.**

***Outcome*: Unwavering resolve.**

Western doctors, Eastern doctors, father-figures and faith collided in one pivotal moment—my body's forceful voice detonating any lingering desire to pursue medicine. I am disappointed but clear. Disillusioned, but free. With kidney yang qi finally unplugged from her "ancestral father line"—and no longer tethered to its purpose and promises—I summon the courage to, once again, egress Dad's path as a clinician and find my own. And so I wonder: *did those tiny purple monks fulfill their promise after all? Have I been ushered home?*

CHAPTER 14

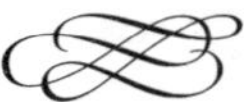

WITH DAVE'S ENCOURAGEMENT, I pick up his camera and never look back. Focusing through a lens, and not the lens of *wellness*, my eyes see, really see, for the first time.

The rapture is immediate. I've never been one to carry a camera, even while traveling abroad, and the intensity of my infatuation surprises me. Before now, cameras felt like a nuisance—interrupting life with their *smile* and *say cheese* solicitations, dragging me out of the moment and into self-consciousness. The delight of losing myself in play was always extinguished by the compulsion to *mark* the moment.

But while my eyes assumed pragmatism, the rest of my body longed for song. Uncertainty and beauty, sorrow and wonder—they had always lived inside me. But without a tool, the poetry of their variance remained buried.

Now, with camera in hand, I am not robbed, but *invited into* the moment. I can finally say what my body is longing to say. Composition, light and Bresson's "decisive moment" reveal the lush, visceral collision within.

One stormy Saturday, fifty-foot swells off the Oregon coast make the news. With Syd at her mom's for the weekend and no other plans, Dave and I grab his camera, hop in the car, and head west. The Sunset Highway ascends into a corridor of Doug Fir, the road lifting us into fog as we listen to his latest mix CD, *Sturgeon Moon* —songs to usher sturgeon, sap and spirit into the dark season. Sigur Ros, Bob Dylan and Magnetic Fields.

When we pull into the sleepy town of Depoe Bay, Dave kills the engine and we watch the sky fall. In Oregon, there are as many kinds of rain as there are days of it. Today, a fine mist wraps around us, but it feels as if it will never really rain, or shower, or drizzle, or pour.

We get out of the car and walk up a steep hill for a better view of the giant waves. Mist shrouds our bodies. From our vantage point, the ocean is a vertical backdrop and the town of Depoe Bay, a theatrical set. The actors have all gone home. The tech crew are turning off the last lights. I feel a terrible, somber ache as the scene unfolds. Loneliness. Heartbreak. Disappointment. Doom. And then the small droplets of mist feel it too—it starts to rain, hard. I tuck the camera under my jacket to wait it out, but Dave runs back to the car to grab an old tee. He knows I need the shot. He always knows what I need before I do.

With his arms and a Nike tee as my shelter, I compose. Adjust. Wait.

Click.

That night, when I open the image on my computer, the melancholy returns. But this time, it comes up for air. And in the surfacing, there is breath, wonder and beauty. I submit the photo to a photography contest and win first place, catalyzing what will become a path of my own, a career in photography.

I begin as a photo assistant at a local studio, shooting primarily weddings, portraits, and some fashion. A stepping stone. I straddle between commercial and documentary photography for a few years, but ultimately, pretty pictures are not enough. I want to see what I feel. And my feelings are found in unedited, unrehearsed, unpolished life. It is here that Dave and I develop a new language together. Ping-ponging images back and forth, we create a photo blog called *XYXX: A visual conversation between two iPhones and two lovers.* Words, our original seduction, evolve into spontaneous, colorful communion. Our megapixel dialogue is more intimate than anything I've ever known.

And so much *fun.*

I am feeling *happy* for the first time in my adult life. Not just fleeting happiness, but something sturdier, something that roots me in the present instead of my body's unraveling. There's a gentle astonishment in it, like discovering a rhythm I never knew was missing. I adore Dave. I'm both enlivened and grounded by our creative, playful intimacy—the antithesis of my navel-gazing past. Around this time, he moves into my home, turning his house into rental—an unceremonious step that feels quietly monumental. Syd's mom has moved far south of Portland, and since Syd is now in high school alongside her sisters down there, the back-and-forth commute is no longer workable. So she stays with us on weekends. In her wonderfully untidy way of moving through the world, she begins planting seeds in me—challenging my need for control, nudging me toward a different way of being: to loosen, to accept, to simply be.

I make a good living working both sides of the camera. I travel a lot, engaging and creating with interesting, accomplished industry folk. I dream into new, bigger projects in both photography and film and bring them to life. There is momentum now, yes—but also an easy delight I had never felt before.

And without realizing it, my body follows. Less hyper-vigilance, fewer spirals of panic. I still have occasional thyroid storms, generalized anxiety, and strange passing-out episodes thanks to my "strong vaso-vagal response." But it's no longer the center of my world. My energy has shifted. Instead of watching my body for signs of betrayal, I am watching the world. And the world, it turns out, is far more interesting than my symptoms.

When I'm working, I don't question this new, creative path. The joy it brings doesn't beg examination. But during restless nights, I still sometimes wonder if I've failed my lineage. *Wasn't I suppose to follow Dad and be a healer? I was born with so much privilege. Am I doing enough to give back? Photos and film don't heal cancer. Am I leaving this world a better place?*

I recall a quote by author, theologian and civil rights leader Howard Thurman, "Don't ask what the world needs. Ask what makes you come alive, and go do it. Because what the world needs is people who have come alive."

But are there limits to this reasoning? Would Howard have praised a daughter's pursuit of art over a more quantifiable, humanitarian service? And yet, art *is* humanitarian, isn't it? Great cinema has repeatedly shaken me out of numbness. Poetry has tapped a forgotten well within. Literature has opened empathic portals to others' experiences. Photographs, paintings, even mixtapes. Art has served me, taught me, helped me to survive.

Medicine is one—sometimes even insufficient—dimension of healing. Is there an entire universe of vitality I've missed? *Is it possible that anything can heal?*

I find myself, semi-consciously, learning to lean into the mystery.

Preparing, perhaps, for my own.

PART III
SELF-IONIZATION

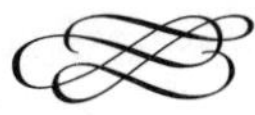

CHAPTER 15

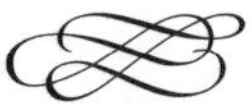

THE BEDROOM WINDOWS are wide open and a cool, Pacific Northwest summer breeze feathers my skin. Morning light reminds closed lids of time and opposites.

Yesterday my friend took her son to swimming lessons at North Portland Rec Center. While her boy flung pre-adolescent limbs through heady chlorine, she snuck into the equipment closet and snapped a few photos of "Timmy and the gang"—plastic, unemployed CPR dummies scattered about in eerie repose, waiting to be rescued. Knowing my affinity for slightly off, dark or storied imagery, my friend texted me the photos that night. We LOL'ed, commented on Timmy's great eyebrows, and then sleep pulled me under. But I nodded off with a curious longing to play with, pose, animate and hold those symbols of resuscitation. I needed them near. I needed to know their story.

In the slack loops between dreaming and waking, I don't open my eyes. Not yet. Images are unfolding:

I see a woman reclining, swimming wrap draped over her body like a burial gown. Poly Blend folds of chemical blue mirror the pool beside her.

I see lifeguards performing rescue drills—mock resuscitation an urgent, red contrast to the woman's ennui.

Compressing 1, 2, 3, 4, 5. Exhale. Exhale.

I see the limbless torso of a CPR mannequin bobbing face-down in the pool.

I fall further into the scene—my body, like a greedy specter, wants every point-of-view.

I feel the quickening rhythm of rescue.

Compressing 1, 2, 3, 4, 5. Exhale. Exhale.

Something startles the woman out of indifference.

She dives in, joining me in the dream state.

Roles blur.

She rescues the mannequin. The savior becomes the saved. The saved, the savior.

Compressing 1, 2, 3, 4, 5. Exhale. Exhale.

A rhythmic then quiet transmutation, ending with the woman face-up on the bottom of the pool.

Un-rescued but alive.

Unsaved but unbound.

Unwavering resolve.

Compressing 1, 2, 3, 4, 5…

INHALE.

She awakens from the dream with a peculiar freedom—no one is coming to save her.

With pictures still playing as I open my eyes, I pull myself from bed, hit rewind, and scribe what I see. But words aren't enough, I want to behold, create, *feel* these images over and over again, like a prayer. Like a film.

MARCH 13, 2014

Dear Charlie,

Mom and I are in Mexico—our mother-daughter Yucatán excursion is over two-decades young. Sometimes family members or friends join but we are the foundation, the shapeless days becoming more so as the arc of our lives align. Once a spring sojourn to honor the anniversary of Dad's death, then a family intervention for Eric's failing marriage, or a yoga intensive—now it's simpler. Lighter. I pack cameras, Mom brings canvases and paint. We talk less, observe more.

This morning while walking the beach—post-café con chocolate-chatty—you entered the conversation. Sometimes, Mom says I remind her of you. Your temperament, your creative pursuits. So I nudged her memory for new details—not in search of any grand revelation, just for the fun of it. An often fruitless endeavor, but today she recalled a picnic you shared just a week after your first encounter. That's a new one. Are there others like this?

After forty years, a forgotten synapse fires and a new scene flickers to life on Mom's mindscape like restored film stock. Will I eventually be able to watch the whole film? Will it be in black-and-white or technicolor? Is it a drama, a comedy or tragedy?

And then—another new detail. A mischievous curandera definitely must have added something extra to the salsa this morning.

Mom plainly revealed, "His full name. I remember it now. Charles Brauer."

CHAPTER 16

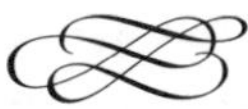

DURING MY LAYOVER IN DENVER, I Google what I know: *Wisconsin Public Access Television. Musician. Charles. Charles Brauer*—in the past, a search without a last name. But today is different. Today, my lifeline crease branches into a million flowering promises.

The album *Blue Sky and Scraped Knuckles* appears on top of my image search. A cyanotype photo of a man kneeling with his dog stares back. His nose is long, eyes gentle. I warm, and bristle, with recognition. *I know that face.*

Dave greets me outside the terminal in Portland with a hug—burnt sugar and cedar envelop and my landing gear settles. For a moment. I intercept our embrace by shoving the saved Google image in Dave's face. I ask with shallow breath and no context, "Who does this look like?" Dave answers without hesitation, "Well I don't know but he looks like he could be your dad."

I search a bit more in the coming weeks but Charles Brauer's web history is strangely sparse, especially for someone with his early achievements. His luddite tendencies from a bygone era help me justify the dearth. *But where is he now? Is he still writing songs, publishing essays and dabbling in television?* I let it go and dismiss my fleeting paternity suspicion as an impossibility. Dad is *Dad* and I haven't reason or bandwidth to think otherwise.

Dave and I are busy writing a new brand initiative for a tech company and planning a photo shoot in Palm Springs. I'm also gearing up for the premiere of my second short film *9* at the Dances With Films festival in Hollywood at the end of May.

Mom suggests I screen my film for her women's group—one of the many circles she's nurtured over the years, each a hearth of mindfulness and friendship. In the film, she plays a wise prima ballerina, crowned with a matted Baba Yaga wig, embodying the gravity of a disfiguring rite of passage with an eerie, unusual elegance. The protagonist, a young ballerina, stumbles upon this secret initiation and must decide how to hold what she's witnessed.

The film begins with a short poem and the opening to Balanchine's *Serenade*, a gestural pose that Balanchine described as "a hymn to ward off the sun."

One ordinary night/ a girl dressed in white /made her mark and faced the dark/ and found it kinder than the light/

The autobiographical nature of the story is uncanny.

When I wrote the script and made the film, however, I had no consciousness of the mother-of-all secrets. Is that why I had my first-ever panic attack before filming? I laid on the living room floor before call time, knees up, feet unable to feel the ground. Like a doula, Mom pressed her reassuring hands onto my arches like I was about to give birth. To what, I didn't know. I was scared of what I could not see.

But the body knows. She always knows. The creative process is mighty mysterious—stories, shapes, and stanzas spring from hidden tunnels in our flesh, beyond reason, beyond understanding. Carl Jung's *A Book of Symbols* often lights my way through these labyrinths, translating *matters of matter* into something my mind can comprehend. Jung states, "A symbol does not define or explain; it points beyond itself to a meaning that is darkly divined yet still beyond our grasp, and cannot be adequately expressed in the familiar words of our language." Worldly objects—from plants, critters, and limbs to mythical beings and cosmic forces—are all part of a lineage of symbolic meaning that the unconscious uses to communicate. I feel, smell, see and hear before I know.

After screening *9* with Mom's gathering in Colorado, the

women reflect, "What was your motivation for making this film?" "What does the secret represent?" We discuss perfectionism, misplaced power, the importance of integrating our shadow selves. We point toward truths but we circle Truth with a capital *T.* We explore secrecy as a concept, but not *the* secret—the one still unformed, unspoken, embryonic. How could we? It remains a seed buried in dark earth—maybe now, just barely stirring, testing if the conditions are right for germination.

This uncertain darkness—not the light or illusion of my conscious self—is a refuge for truth and harbinger of my becoming.

At the end of the film, Baba Yaga stands before the young ballerina with her severed big toe—her broken, fallible humanity no longer a secret. But the girl doesn't run. She relaxes. Mirroring each other, they begin Balanchine's *Serenade* again, but this time, whole.

Sensing the rising temperature, the first offering of spring rain in the soil, the seed coat gets ready to break open.

CHAPTER 17

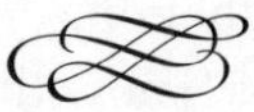

ANOTHER AIRPORT GIVES rise to curiosity, to Googling. While waiting for my flight home from my film screening, I dial the University of Wisconsin Madison's library where Charles Brauer's album was produced. I'm following a thin trail of bread crumbs, just for the fun of it, a casual detour, nothing serious. *Life is mysterious, don't take it so serious.*

But as I wait for someone to answer, a flicker of something unnamed tightens in my chest. The fantasy isn't harmless. It's a door I can't afford to open. A mysterious man at the end of the trail, open arms, a knowing smile. I let the image form for the briefest moment—too long—before I heave it back into the dark where it belongs.

A helpful student answers my call. When asked about the album, she replies, "Nothing off the top of my head rings a bell, but I have a long evening ahead and would be happy to do some digging for you."

Wasted bread. I let it go, fly home and turn in. I have a week of early call times ahead and need to put my sleuthing to rest.

But early the next morning, I receive an email from Farrah McDaniel.

Subject: Information Regarding Charles Brauer

Dear Kimberly,

My name is Farrah and I was the library student you spoke to over the phone last night about Charles Brauer. As promised, I continued to do some more digging for information about Charles' life and I'm pretty certain I found something. During my search I came across an article in the Milwaukee Journal dated Wednesday, October 2, 1985 about a missing sailor by the name of Charles Brauer whose boat was found washed-ashore in Sturgeon Bay, Wisconsin. I was about to dismiss it until I read that during the 1970's Charles hosted a history-oriented series for the Wisconsin Educational Television Network, which included traveling with his dog, Ranger, a banjo and a guitar. I received further confirmation when I read that he had recently finished building a home in Ferryville, WI, where his records were also published.

I need to drive to work. But the car keys in my hand suddenly feel funny—weightless, insubstantial—sensory signals interrupted by my brainstem sounding alarm. My diaphragm retreats to higher ground. I sense danger is near.

I spend the next five days in an internet fire-walled studio, my impulsive tendencies tamed by a corporate muzzle. But once home, the beast is free and she howls under the blue glow of my screen. I'm glued to my task like an addict at a slot machine, waiting for the right combination of Google search words to bring me back to certainty, to safety. But information on Charlie's disappearance is piecemeal. One news source posts his obituary. *He's dead?* Another says his body was never found. *He's missing, not dead?* I research the surviving family members and find more crumbs—a sister with oil-pastel paintings in a Grand Haven gallery, a filmmaker brother from Traverse City. I pull up the filmmaker's profile on Facebook and scroll through pictures of his children. I zoom in on their faces and ask their features to complete me. *Are you my cousins? What do you love? Is that my nose?*

Each new bit of data lands in my cells like a tiny electrical storm—impatient, ungrounded, building in strength and intensity. I don't know where or how to find shelter.

* * *

On Saturday Dave and I are eager to throw off the week's stress with a spring bike ride along Portland's waterfront. A twenty-five mile loop on single-speed bikes, the monotony of rubber-on-concrete has become a welcome, if seasonal, ritual for us—four spinning prayer wheels quieting the noise in our heads. Before reaching the waterfront trail, we navigate a few neighborhood streets and then a long stretch on Naito Parkway. It's a relatively quiet street, mostly lined with trees and residential parking. Dave and I ride in single file, but I keep close, enjoying his occasional tail wag that says, *We're in this together.*

I do not see the car door's violent kiss. I do not feel my sudden weightlessness or the pavement that follows. I only hear a voice, *my* voice—unwilled, guttural, coarse, and then the sound of my helmet cracking. I lay in the street wondering, *Will we still grill burgers tonight?*

As endorphins try to sort out a plan, linear time tangles into a tight, matted ball. Bits of asphalt puncture moments into my flesh—

I hear a young woman behind me. She's on the phone with her dad, pacing. Clouds above accumulate. The blue behind them, unsure. A young massage student with kind eyes approaches. He offers me a few free sessions. Dave is near but not near enough, his voice in stereo, over there, then over there. The sky is more blue than grey. No, more grey than blue. The young woman approaches. Her eyes aren't kind. She offers her hand, but to introduce herself, not to help me up off the pavement. My low-angled hand-shake feels silly. Someone tells me to move out of the road. The clouds build, I try on their confidence, but grey wins.

When an ambulance arrives, an EMT prepares a shot of pain medication for the ride. "No thanks," I say, feeling nothing—dope-happy on my own internal pharmacy. But when the vehicle takes a hard left turn, I yowl. The EMT laughs, asks again and I oblige. When reality turns into a sweet, distant syrup, I hear Dave's voice under the blaring siren. *Dave! There you are! Are you OK?* He doesn't hear my silent call, so I exit my skin to sit shotgun on his lap.

The driver calls out, "Need a vomit bag up here." But other than asphalt studded hands and a belly full of worry and adrenaline, Dave's okay. He'd flown over his bike too—not from the car door, but from the sound of my impact, the sudden jolt of realization. I was behind him when it happened. He must have slammed his brakes the moment he heard me hit, his body reacting faster than his mind could catch up.

Together, we were right-side up in the upside down. But time and circumstance want to test this delicate balance.

CHAPTER 18

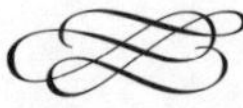

After two fentanyl-filled days at the hospital, I return home with a five-inch pelvic fracture and six weeks of bed rest ahead. But prescribed stillness for bone healing can't mend what I don't yet know is breaking. Beneath the surface—quiet, insistent, unnoticed even by me—something has started to sunder. A fault line threading through my identity, carving its way forward before I'm ready to feel it.

The over-stuffed living room sofa becomes my bed. Cushions sag and curdle under my body. Days mush into one another. *Horror vacui* inspires obnoxious, Sharpie-red circles in my calendar marking time with X-rays and follow-ups. I can't sit, only recline—any weight on my pelvic bone could shift the non-displaced fracture and send me into surgery. Plus, it kills to sit. Time doesn't care how many brushstrokes she takes to complete her painting. I am either an irritable bystander watching her sweeping gestures, or I can choose to become the gesture. I give in. I eat, sleep and stare at the safety-orange chandelier on the ceiling. Once upon a time, I thought this homemade light fixture was cool, an emblem of my budding interest in visual arts. It takes only a few horizontal days to realize it's not cool. Or art.

During the first few weeks, I think about Charlie. I have more than enough time now to bloodhound his—my?— mystery. But the hunt unsettles me—a deep vibration within, constant and electric, like hyperthyroid tremors that won't still, even with 24/7 bedrest. I try to go slowly but am haunted by the scent of my own blood near. When I receive an email from Wisconsin Public Television—a response to a dozen random inquiries sent and forgotten—I open a link titled, *Hunters on Wings*, with host Charles Brauer, and watch the twelve-minute segment. Tectonic plates shift within my psyche; a thin fissure forms. The timbre in his voice, familiar. His stature, my own. I dismiss what I see *(I must!)* as confirmation bias: a mind seeking to confirm what it already suspects. But then there it is, and as unsentimental as it gets. Charlie crouches on the ground, a close-up of his hands pointing at meadow vole droppings. Those. Are. Undeniably. My. Hands. Mom, Dad and Eric all have stubby nail beds, average-length and straight-as-arrow fingers. I have long nail beds, long fingers and crooked pinkies. So does Charlie.

Fear compresses my ego's geology. The fault widens and I teeter on its edge. To save myself, I put the bloodhound back in his crate.

Instead, I cling to the known, to a narrative with more answers than questions. Bone fracture healing occurs in three distinct but overlapping stages: the early inflammatory stage (first 2 weeks), the repair stage (6 weeks), and the late remodeling stage in which the healing bone is restored to its original shape, structure, and mechanical strength. Fibroblasts and osteoblasts in my pelvis are already connecting broken ends and forming new bone. I will be walking again before summer's end. That's a nice, tidy timeline. It feels good to know, to sturdy myself with understanding and finitude.

When I look at my x-rays, I see a lightning bolt crack running nearly the entire length of my foundation. I grasp for metaphor: a fissure of magic leading to other realities, beyond earthly boundaries, like a crack in time. Or the reverse—the light in Georgia O'Keeffe's *Dark Abstraction* suggesting spirit pressing into matter, entering the dense world through a fracture. A new day arrives at the crack of dawn, a gateway between night and day, where mythic heroes descend into the underworld and prayers rise toward heaven. Or, as Leonard Cohen sings, *"There is a crack in everything, that's how the light gets in."*

This is the narrative I can get behind.

So with time on my side, I devote hours to an inward, anatomical regard. And more specifically, the pelvis. *What an elegant and expressive mass of bone! The reaching span of iliac wings! The bowl shaped acetabulum that allows the femur head to rotate with less than one-tenth the friction of ice on ice! The sacral bone that whimsically joins both wings into the caricature of a butterfly!*

I cling to a vision of my new wings brimming with magic—my own matter penetrated by light, a promise of renewal, a metamorphosis underway.

But even a butterfly can sense early seismic activity. I steady myself with metaphor and meaning while an abyss readies to open greedy and wide beneath my feet.

CHAPTER 19

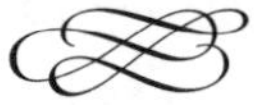

Seven weeks later, Dave and I deliver my crutches to Goodwill. One foot in front of the other, bones consent to gravity, but I'm afraid. The center of my body feels fragile—a primal din unnoticed (ignored?) until the animal's cage broke. I feel timid. Protective. Dave and I are emotionally worn too. During bedrest, I was one-too-many-dependents for a father already carrying the weight of a daughter who, by summer, had officially aged out of the public education system—a milestone that didn't mark independence, but rather, the beginning of lifelong uncertainty. The question *"What's next?"* looms. We try to regain normalcy, but while bones healed, tectonic plates continued to grind and shove under stress. I start swimming laps at the Nike pool. The repetition and linear task of flesh-dividing-water help me gain strength and control over other, less effortless divides.

We travel to Colorado early August to visit family. Despite being upright and walking again, something hasn't rooted; tentative limbs reach but do not grab. I retreat from Colorado's dry, too-sunny expanse into the pool—a fluid balm for instability. Submerged, there is nothing to hold onto, nothing to steady or unsteady me. Water joins me in ambiguity.

Our first morning, while Dave and family stitch invisible loops between espresso maker, bathroom, and fridge, I go outside for a swim. I use the word "swim" lightly because today, I spend the majority of time bobbing up and down, mostly down. It's not enough to feel water briefly splash across my face. I want full immersion. I sit on the bottom of the shallow end, legs crossed, and let water's body move my body until we are one. I want to be rippled sand on the floor of Lake Winnebago. I want to be smooth rock in Lake Michigan's great depths. I need to feel home again because up there on solid earth, I've lost my ground.

Eventually thoughts of *something salty, something crunchy*, pull me from my underworld. Food and hunger never fail to tether me to reality. I grab a handful of potato chips, and wander around the house looking for Eric. I need to orbit in big brother warmth. I'm not the only one who feels good in Eric's presence; his Viking stature is dwarfed by unparalleled presence and heart. I get an extra dose because he's making up for my childhood of Spock bites, gleeking, and Guantanamo Barbie.

I find him sitting in his office behind an inconceivable stack of stuff. Still wrapped in a wet towel, I move a pile and replace it with my butt. Despite the clutter, I always feel calm and safe in his spaces—his office, garage, and the elaborate Faraday cage/bomb shelter he built are all architectural proxies for his good hugs.

"Hey, I got something for you," he says while opening a drawer. I smile, not knowing what it is, but return to a countless string of unprompted, big-brother gifts from the past: the Rubbermaid toolbox filled with every handy gadget an unhandy girl might need, the protective amulet for my solo European travels, the tactical hair clip for MacGyver-ing myself out of danger. In an apocalypse, Eric will keep me safe.

He hands me a small 5" x 5" box with a bright graphic on its cover. It reads, *Welcome to you.*

I know what it is. The apocalypse might be sooner than anticipated.

"Hey, J and I have been messing around with our DNA test results lately. Thought you'd want in on the fun, so I got you a kit."

Subtext: *Who's your daddy?*

Sub-subtext: But really, what are the chances?

"Gulp," One deceptively simple syllable for the narrative it writes in my gut.

Eric grins, punching my arm. "For my sister-from-another-mister,"

"Har har." I roll my eyes. "Honestly, what are the odds? I'm more likely the product of immaculate conception than of Mom's one-night fling."

Eric smirks, "Well Mom *did* report having her first sexual fantasy about Jesus."

"That tracks."

"The only real mystery," I say, shaking the box, "is why Dad only gave *me* the smart gene."

"Touché."

We let the joke land where it always has—on the surface, light. A harmless rib at Mom's Free Love chapter, a family artifact we dust off for our amusement. We laugh only because we know it's not true.

The bloodhound has been put down. He was a good boy.

I turn the box over in my hands—along the edge, candy-colored chromosomes belie the box's Pandoric powers. Holding the box that will bomb the joke into silence—once and for all—sends a deep taproot down, through my pruned toes, and into the earth for the first time since the week of the accident.

But unpacking it from my suitcase a week later, the kit no longer resembles a harmless box of Mike & Ikes. I stash it in the medicine cabinet, hiding it behind a large tub of chewable Vitamin C. I don't want to see it every time I take my vitamins. I tell myself, *Wait a while, take the test casually, maybe after a glass of wine or when I've completely forgotten about it. It's no big deal. It will just confirm what I've already known for nearly forty years. Dad is Dad. Duh!*

An hour later, I march right back into the kitchen, open up the box and spit into a tube.

I receive an email from 23andMe five weeks later; my genetic results are in, including DNA relatives and a basic genetic profile. I open the link and briefly scan a colorful map (more friendliness! So fun! So harmless!) with my European ancestry composition. No surprises other than some Ashkenazi Jewish ancestry that might explain the Israelson surname on Mom's side. Then I open DNA relatives. Eric Warner is at the top. We share 22% of our DNA segments. That's a lot! That's good! See? He's my brother. So what if we have different nailbeds.

But I read more closely. According to 23andMe, 22% isn't enough to make him my full brother. Right next to his name, the name I have known for 39 years as my big brother, I read:

Eric Warner: Half-Sibling

* * *

I tell Dave first. I need his body, his surety, his gravity. For as long as I can remember, I'm more stable in the world when I'm physically attached, flesh-on-flesh, to sentient life. As a kid, Mom and Dad were my hosts, arm or hip pressed parasitically into them. In junior high, when I learned this behavior wasn't cool or even acceptable, I became a psychic barnacle, orbiting the space of anyone or anything safe and solid. With the roots of a giant Doug Fir, Dave is my lightening rod, my earthing system, my infinite sink for excess charge.

I sit next to him on the bed until he stirs. His lids are heavy with sleep but they register my presence. I roll over on top of him (I'm going to need full-body grounding this time) and wait until he's alert enough to comprehend me. I don't want to have to say it twice.

"Eric is my half-brother." I say it calmly. Dead pan. I'm a terrible actress. When I feel overwhelmed, I go flat. Or worse, emotionally inappropriate, as if my brain blows a circuit, signals all crisscross-applesauce. The corners of my mouth sneak up, ready to crack. My ribcage vibrates, tamping down uncontrollable laughter.

Dave doesn't say anything. What is there to say? In his head, lights are going on. Puzzle pieces are flying into place. His gut always sensed "something off" about my place in the Warner clan. He pulls me close. I want to stay in his arms forever. As long as my head is pressed against his chest, I don't need to do anything with this news. But even with the slow rhythm of his heartbeat, my thoughts travel in a thousand unfinished directions. *Did Dad know... Did Mom...How could I not know...Did I know? What do I call Dad now...*

What do I call this is other man…this Charlie? And can we even be certain he's my father?

I look in the mirror and study my face; I brush my teeth; make a fried egg on toast; feed Kitty Pang—everyday routines but now someone else is doing them. I don't know how to integrate the results so I don't. By that evening, survival strategies take over and I convince myself it's a mistake. Denial, alongside magical-thinking—my sweet, anesthetizing friends.

I reach out to 23andMe for clarification. Corroboration.

Dear 23andMe,

Please interpret my DNA data. I share 22% DNA with my brother. Is this on a sliding scale? Could it still indicate a full sibling relationship? Could we have the same parents but just share a little less DNA than other siblings? What if my DNA was contaminated? How accurate is your data? Was my sample accidentally dropped? Did 38% of my DNA land on the floor, the other half of my half-sibling relationship forever lost in a biohazard dumpster somewhere? Can I get it back?

I fall asleep tallying, grasping, clinging.

Eric and I are both tall. We're both ashy blond. I'm hairy, he's harrier. We both like poetry. But he prefers action films; I like psychological horror. I throw things away. He holds on. I like the company of one. He likes the company of many. Dad was tall. Mom says I have Dad's legs, his lower lip. We both loved science. But Dad was fair-skinned, and I'm olive. Dad leaned toward depression; I lean toward anxiousness. Dad found boundaries confining; for me, they comfort.

I open a reply from 23andMe the next morning. It's confirmed: 22% is not enough shared DNA to be full-blooded siblings. I screen grab the original result—**Eric Warner: Half Sibling**—and text it to Mom and Eric.

Their replies reach another recipient. She reads their responses. She answers when they call. She registers their genuine shock and concern. She hears Mom insist there were no other flings, only Charlie. She hears reassurances of steadfast love. But I'm too far away to get the message.

Pathways for dissociation are already primed. One lane whispers, "This is scary. Proceed slowly. Find your feet, find your feelings." The other shouts, "I think I can, I think I can." The latter is bold, impulsive, ready to forge ahead with this new information. Ready to walk on coals. Brave positivity with a glittering bow-on-top.

But in the dark den of cellular oblivion, someone else stirs—a lioness twitches her paws in a fitful, apocalyptic dream. Sensing a truth far more dangerous than pretty, she stays in hiding. I try to convince myself it's no big deal. Nothing has changed. And the truth is, nothing has changed. But my insides don't agree and logic can't talk them out of it.

My body goes silent. Cell metabolism slows, preparing itself for a long winter. My nervous system responds in the only way it knows how—popsicle. Outwardly, I share the story with manic excitement. People encourage me to share, write the story down, turn it into a film. *It's wild! It's beautiful! It's meaningful! I think I can, I think I can!* My stomach says rest, but I don't. My nerves say slow down, but I can't. I compulsively continue to share the story with everyone who'll listen, trying it on like a new pair of stiff denim and each time, wishing them relaxed and full of holes.

It's unnerving to realize they're the best fit I've ever owned.

CHAPTER 20

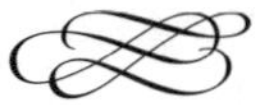

Dave and I travel to Wisconsin in September. Autumn is an especially colorful time to visit the Midwest and we'd wanted to make the trip for years. With careful planning around Syd's care schedule, we carve out a week just for us—a rare stretch of time to step away, to breathe.

During my six weeks on Planet Sofa (and pre-DNA revelation), my bare feet itched to touch familiar ground, and the ground I needed was rich, loamy soil fed by cycles of corn and wheat, thunder and snow. I'd close my eyes and traverse her fields, the thick smell of bovine nectar descending me down, down, down into solid, unfailing earth. I killed time looking for VRBOs and after finding a tiny red cottage on Fire Lane 13, just a shoreline-mile from my childhood home, I booked a trip.

We arrive in Milwaukee late in the month and drive north on Hwy 43 (yes, *that* one) to Two Rivers. I want Dave to see Lake Michigan before we head inland and Two Rivers is on the lake's western border. Our first rental is modest and tidy and an unexpected Monarch butterfly migration jazzes up its propriety. The first morning I step outside the door to a conifer-shaped kaleidoscope of black and orange. So while Dave sits at the kitchen table wrapping up a brand deck, I spend an absurd amount of time shaking the tree's branches and then standing inside the winged blaze. Butterflies make metamorphosis look fun and I'm grateful for their reassurance.

That night, I slide open the long, east-facing windows of our bedroom—placed just high enough up the wall to obscure the highway so while horizontal, all I see is Lake Michigan. Good enough for me. I listen to crickets until the lake's long, rhythmic licks lull me to sleep. Unguarded, the Midwest pour herself into me.

At 2:00am, I roll over, floating upwards into brain waves just shallow enough to detect a subtle flash of light in the room. I open my eyes and look out over Lake Michigan. Everything is silent. No crack of thunder, no more crickets—just a quiet, undulating wave of heat lightning straddling the horizon. I adjust my pillow and watch the show.

Without the slightest foresight, I had booked this rental on the anniversary of Charles Brauer's disappearance.

September 23, 1985, my *biological father*—the words feel like a foreign language— hopped aboard his beloved sailboat Fogbow in Frankfurt, Michigan. He was headed across the lake, a routine passage to Sturgeon Bay, Wisconsin. An expert sailor—intimately familiar with Lake Michigan's late summer temperament—he had navigated this route successfully hundreds of times. Just a month before his disappearance, he published an article in *Sailing Magazine*, warning fellow sailors of the season's treachery. He had written, "but if you want things like home, then stay home."

So true to his nature, he set sail into the lake's unpredictable season.

That night a historic storm came up over the lake and washed Fogbow thirty-five feet ashore, just north of Sturgeon Bay.

Charles was never found.

Twenty-nine years ago—*to the day*—I could've looked out these very windows (just down shore from Sturgeon Bay) to see Fogbow and the giant swells overtaking its deck. With a strong pair of binoculars, maybe I could've even seen Charlie's struggle.

I map out our overlapping, multi-dimensional timelines—the serendipitous timing and location is uncanny—and I begin to feel a strange sense of being guided along in a story that has already been written. My inner rainbow-studded-unicorn has always wanted to experience magic and now the universe is dumping bags full of glitter on my head.

The next morning I say hi to my new winged friends before crossing the highway to a narrow beach. A few hitchhikers flutter around my head as I descend off the bank onto rocky sand. I throw off my shoes and kneel; I splash my face with cold lake water and picture Charlie's DNA joining mine—a double-helix hug from my paternal line. I try to feel new roots stretching from my recently healed pelvis into his fluid tomb. *Are fragments of his bones under my bare toes? What were his last moments, his last thoughts?*

Or *were* they his last? *His boat was found but never his body.* How is that possible? It's a giant lake but don't bodies float after drowning?

Later that morning, while Dave navigates us to the tip of Wisconsin's thumb, I dig into an uplifting Google search "Do corpses float?" Turns out, yes. If the earth ever floods, we will eventually return to the light of day, blue, bloated and gassy. Initially, bodies sink but as they decompose and bacteria inflates us like a balloon, we rise like the living dead. *So if this is true, Charlie would've been found, right? It's not the ocean after all.* But I'm not convinced so I return to Professor Google. "Do Lake Michigan corpses float?"

Aha. Lake Michigan is an exception to the rule. Considered the deadliest of the Great Lakes, this body of water is home to more shipping disasters—those involving large loss of life—than all the other Great Lakes combined. The lake's distinctive longitudinal shape, running 307 miles from north to south, with almost unbroken shores on either side, make it vulnerable to sudden shifts in weather patterns. Sailors can find themselves setting sail in the morning on a clear, blue sky day and meeting eighteen-foot swells that evening. And it's deep. Too cold and deep for natural decomposition. Sometimes referred to as an icy graveyard, Lake Michigan's bottom is littered with mummified bodies, resting-in-peace for hundreds of years.

I put my phone down and close my eyes. I understand why humans build burial sites. Grief is a vacuum and we anchor ourselves against its pull with heavy, conclusive tombstones. Or flowering plums. Our void needs a place to go. I've found comfort over the years swimming in Winnebago and imagining Dad's ashes swirling around me like stardust. Or when I'm not there, dancing with sturgeon. *Dancing.* His wish for me.

But the image of my other father, shipwrecked, mummified in cold, desolate deep—this one is hard for me. And grieving someone I never knew feels wrong, indulgent, misplaced. There's nowhere to put this black hole. No lake, no stone, no sky. So I fall into its singularity, reaching the limits of grief, collapsing in on itself and consumed into a cloud of nothingness.

Burial at Sea

A young boy
beachsand dried to ankles
finds a dead gull washed ashore
and
holding quiet weight
and
feeling stiff satin plumage
resolves
Burial at Sea
  So
while oars in old locks
creak probable gull-tones
the mourned
  carefully placed on the back seat
glides
just above calm blue waters
  only now
  wings tucked
  eyes closed
  feet bound to a round rock
Well off shore
the young boy
halts the boat to
listen
to
hear
  water gurgle beneath wooden strakes
  Come, come home
  Come, come home
Clenched innocent hands
relax around splintery oars
to move
lightly
the weighted bird
    over the edge
   to hold

a long moment upon the surface
eternity
  this matter of natural balanced fact
    then
      Releases
      and wide-eye watches
    the World
  too, too rapidly
sink
almost from view
to where
  in blue-green ripple
    and sun-streak distortion
       Sudden great wings unfold
         reach out
           to fly
             a new
               soft
              spiral
            wonderfully
          silent
        away

- Charles Brauer

OCTOBER 1, 2014

Dear Charlie,

Just seven years after publishing your poem Burial At Sea / holding quiet weight / and / feeling stiff satin plumage / resolves / Burial at Sea / you also stretched great wings to fly their / new, soft spiral / wonderfully silent / away.

When you were on water, did she speak of your looming death? Was she your playmate, your lover or foe? Are we drawn to elements that eventually undraw us?

I think about what it must have been like to sink into great depths, to see a bottomless eternity below and feel your weight drawn into it. Did you feel pulled? Or did you soar, like the gull, wingless sails outstretched to guide you somewhere beyond?

Are your bones still at the bottom? Were they ever?

I'm still in Wisconsin. Dave and I were supposed to fly back to Oregon today but a fire started at O'hare airport and our connecting flight was canceled. Instead of wasting a day with airline agents, we rode serendipity and spent an extra vacation day exploring Milwaukee. I especially wanted to visit the Wisconsin Historical Society and learn more about you. We scoured the data base and found articles on the accident, your high-school paperboy band, a few old pamphlets announcing live readings and music gigs. I found a bit on your television series Long Ago Is All Around, which you proudly claimed as "the number one show in nursing homes." I'd give my left pinky toe to know if you were bragging or meant that as a joke. I also learned that, as one newspaper wrote, you have a "special way with children" and alongside your co-host coon-hound Ranger, performed gigs at Wisconsin elementary schools teaching poetry and history through song.

Did you ever visit my school?

Would you have recognized yourself in the pig-tailed girl singing along enthusiastically in the front row? Would you have been irritated or amused if she threw herself on Ranger and wouldn't let go?

CHAPTER 21

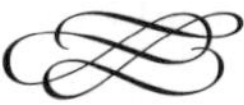

Researching Charlie is a welcome distraction for the restless, homeless emotions inside me. Sleuthing gives sadness a temporary place to land. But after a few hours at the library, Dave and I have exhausted our search. I'm not satisfied. An unsettling mystery surrounds Charlie's death, but I sense it lived in him long before—woven into his creative voice and the maverick spark that fueled him. I need more. His story is fractured, piecemeal, like an old film-strip with too many missing frames. I keep waiting for the full picture to emerge, but all I get is flickering light, glimpses of a life half-seen, half-lost.

Upon returning to Portland I decide to reach out to Charlie's siblings. They may have some of those frames. They may also want to know their beloved brother left a part of himself behind. They may also *not* want to know.

I craft a letter, writing my way through shock and emotion. I am not 100% sure I will send it, but my words on the screen make it real. And possible. Deep freeze and auto-pilot coexist in my nervous system, an uneasy alliance that keeps me moving before true catatonia can set in. I am no longer thinking clearly; instead, I let the momentum of life hurl me into the maelstrom of uncertainty that is now home.

I have to send it. My life depends on it.

I hit COMMAND P, fold the paper carefully and stuff it in an envelope. I seal my fate with a Forever stamp.

October 2, 2014

Dear Richard,

I'm not quite sure how to write this letter, so forgive me if I stumble. I think it's best I just jump right in.

When I was 17, my mom took me for a long walk along the NE shoreline of Lake Winnebago and told me there was a question about my paternity. She had met your brother, Charles Brauer, at the Mariposa Festival in Canada on the summer solstice of 1974. They shared an evening together. She was already a few weeks pregnant—or so she believed—so she and my dad never questioned my paternity. And, without access to DNA tests or easy internet searches, neither did I.

My father was my father in every way that mattered, and when he died suddenly in a car accident a half-year later, that truth only solidified. Eventually, I forgot all about it.

But this past spring, while walking with my mom on a beach in Mexico, she shared more details—his last name, his creative pursuits. When I returned home, curiosity led me to Google, where I found Charles' albums and old TV segments. Seeing his face, hearing his voice, watching his hands move—sent me reeling.

Then, I took a DNA test with my brother Eric. When the results came back confirming we were half-siblings, I found myself logging in daily, rechecking in disbelief.

Now, of course, anyone in their right mind would probably be a bit incredulous of this story. And I completely understand these feelings. I, myself, am needing to move cautiously and am also open to the possibility of error. For all I know, I may even have the wrong brother Richard and if this is the case, please use this letter as inspiration on your next screenplay or a good laugh with your production crew.

I do know my mother wasn't with anyone else other than my father during the time of my conception and that there is no question around my brother's paternity.

I also know this letter is probably very difficult and maybe even painful to receive. I can only imagine what it would be like to lose a loving, free-spirited brother many years ago, then, decades later, learn that part of him might still live on. Please know that I come to you with no expectations. I simply feel that if the roles were reversed, I would want to know. I just have a simple yearning to know more about Charles—his life, his passions, the parts of him I may unknowingly carry forward.

I've lived with this mystery my whole life and I can continue to do so. So if you choose not to reply, I completely respect your wishes and privacy (and the rest of your family's) and you will never hear from me again. And if you do decide to connect, well… that could be a very sweet and strange homecoming for us all.

I would be happy to share my online DNA profile with you if you need confirmation and want to do your own test. You can also find me on all the normal social networking sites under Kimberly Warner in case you need to assuage some part of you that worries I'm some sort of lunatic.

And again, if I've found the wrong Richard, please accept my apologies. My partner Dave and I just returned from a late summer holiday in Wisconsin to spend time with Lake Michigan and Winnebago and say hello to the magnificent midwestern season in transition. We also enjoyed a few hours at the Milwaukee Historical Society and found some newspaper clippings on Charles' performances and the WPT television show *Long Ago is All Around*. And I suppose that title about sums it up for me. In pursuing more information about Charles' life long ago, I hope my present life can be a more intimate and informed celebration of the man who unknowingly shared his passion and spirit with a daughter.

I hope this finds you with a smile.

Sincerely,

Kimberly

* * *

I wait, rising each morning with an impatient, singular focus—*check email*. But weeks pass. Notifications disappoint and my dopamine receptors eventually look elsewhere for more fulfilling, reliable hits. I thicken my skin and prepare to hear nothing from the Brauers, or worse, a resounding "Leave us alone." I have no idea what to expect so I try my hardest to expect nothing.

I turn back to research, something I can control. The inner hound I put down after Eric gave me the DNA kit has been resurrected, tracking clues that lead to the most vulnerable prey of all—my own identity. And all the while, the other parts of my identity recede out of focus; I had spent so much of life laser chasing answers about my physical health, my lack of it, the mystery of why my body does the things it does—but now, *now* there is another mystery. My ever-changing, ever-puzzling symptoms seem to swim away, making room for all-things-Charlie.

I learn that before his disappearance, Charlie had just finished hand-building a two-story home in rural Ferryville, Wisconsin. On the mailbox, not far from the Mississippi River, he painted his name —Charles Brauer—followed by an insistent declaration: *Home and Away*. According to one journalist, he liked to say "That's where you'll find me—home, or away." *Way to commit, Dad.* I Google Map the location and make a mental note to visit it someday.

I also email an acquaintance of Mom's—a well-known harpist who, on occasion, spoke about Charlie and their friends-with-benefits relationship. Turns out, he had a lot of girlfriends. Often, at the same time.

She shares: "I heard about his death long after the fact and was shocked and saddened. I never told this to anyone before but I harbored a secret fantasy that he had staged the sailing accident to fake his death and was living happily ever after with his girlfriend across the lake who inherited his life insurance policy. As farfetched as it seemed, at the time it made more sense than imagining the senseless death of someone so young and talented. I'm not sure his girlfriend(s) knew about each other but he was very handsome, charismatic and hard to resist, as your mother can attest. Beside all his obvious charms, he was a very soulful and tender person, a man's man with a poet's heart."

I ignore "faked his death" and the sandwiched "s" after girlfriend and instead I hold onto "soulful" and "poet."

Why do I need him to be good? What if he was a philandering misogynist?

What if he staged his death for insurance money? Would it make a difference? Did he marry? What was he like in relationship? Was he kind?

Short of trying to locate his little black book, I decide the second best way to learn about Charlie's heart is through his music. I order all three of his albums on eBay and study each one carefully, dutifully—the cover art, inserts, graphics, band members, and most of all, his lyrics.

The self-produced albums are a blend of folk and bluegrass with a hint of goofball. A multi-talented instrumentalist, he accompanies himself on guitar, banjo, harmonica or jaw harp, and sometimes it seems, all at once. I dissect his lyrics, trying to decipher my own genetic code. Ranging from heartfelt and personal to lively, regional ballads peppered here and there with poetry, the albums are as close as I may ever get to not just feeling my biological father near, but knowing his soul.

I study, listen, let his voice, lilt and intention fall into me:

From the poem "The Blanket" I'm reminded of the quiet comfort of strangers I feel when traveling, a surrendering together: */ A thick blanket of random humanity / bordered by the silk of implicit trust /*

And the song "Attic Window" mirrors my own love of solitude: */ I'd love to go there when it rained / just to sit and look outside / you could hear the rain upon the roof / and feel so satisfied*

His lively "Redbone Coonhound", an ode to Ranger, reflects my own enthusiasm for all things covered in fur: */ riding in my truck or walking by my side / I swear that old hound is a friend of mine / in the middle of the night when I can't sleep / we'll go out together looking for coons on the street /*

And "Birtha", the one that makes me want to weep and be the stray that accompanies his loneliness: */ we sat down together the cat and me / won't forget the night she was a friend don't you see / it was my birthday and nobody came / except a black and white cat without any name*

Through song and poetry, a 2-dimensional snapshot of Charlie begins to move and breathe; he grows a beating heart with longing, preferences, humor and hope. He is a creative spirit, a wanderer. He doesn't like being boxed-in or labeled. He prefers solitude. He scorns city life and romanticizes the past. I feel so much resonance, like an echo finally returning after a lifetime of waiting.

I know that man. He is the stranger I've known forever, living inside of me.

Or was I a stranger living inside of him? His banjo tune "Have you Seen" hauntingly sings out *yes.*

In the chorus, Charlie pleas— / *Oh have you seen my love of two years / since we parted company / I fear that she is carrying our child / our child that never will be / [...] / though in my mind it is the best for all / though my heart says no let's wait and see / to think I'm the father of a daughter or a son / and to know that it never will be.*

Love of two years? Either Charlie is taking poetic liberties with lyrics, Mom is a great historical revisionist, or I have another half-sibling(s?) out there. Whatever the truth may be, it's clear that he felt *something.* He intuited his own flesh and blood was roaming the planet, enough so that he wrote a song about it. The line "to know that it never will be" puzzles me though. How could he be so certain? Was he reflecting on his own desire (or lack-thereof) to be a father? Or was the mother in a situation she couldn't escape?

Or is it something more, a sense that his own life would end too soon, that when the truth finally surfaced, he would already be long gone?

CHAPTER 22

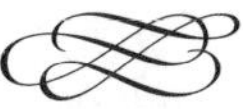

ON HALLOWEEN, when a thin veil separates the living and the dead, I receive an email from Richard Brauer.

Kimberly,

Amazing! I received your letter thinking that it must be something related to an event I was working on. You can imagine my jaw dropping silence, turning to a smile as I read further. It is truly a wonderful thing that you mustered the courage to contact me. I was 30 when Chuck vanished on Lake Michigan on September 23, 1985. There is a plaque on a park bench in Frankfort honoring him. 3 healthy Red Maples flank the bench.

It took a couple weeks to share your letter with my sisters, Janet and Carol, since I knew we were getting together. I copied your letter and let them read it as I watched. It was an unforgettable experience. They are also thrilled and will surely be contacting you.

I'm going to keep this short for now, but wanted to let you know that we are excited to meet you and your mom and share the zillion stories about Charles, known to us as Chuck. He was an adventurous spirit!!!

BTW, you have 9 cousins here!!! Ages 28–45 I think. My kids are the youngest of the group.

Words hardly express the excitement.

Welcome.

Rich

Ps: Attached is a photo I took of Chuck in 1972 with his new pup Ranger.

Welcome. This simple, pedestrian word has never. In my life. Meant more. Than it does now. Seven letters strung together, long and round, are gentle arms. I am welcome. I read the letter again. And again. Rich's words embrace and nudge me down onto solid ground. But the ground is quicksand. I am overwhelmed. Excited. Anxious. It is real now and I can't erase what I've done. There. Is. No. Turning. Back.

I stare at the attached black and white portrait of Charlie and Ranger. *Chuck* and Ranger. He is just twenty-three in the photo. His shoulders are broad and I fixate on the way his torso cradles Ranger, the good boy who accompanies him everywhere, on stage, in the woods and even has a barking cameo on an album. I am envious of Ranger, longing to feel the weight of myself in this man's arms. *What would it be like? Would I feel safe? Would my body anchor in our shared, unquestioning blood?* I title a new folder on my desktop "Charlie," and drag the photo in. Like a girl with a grade-school crush, I make it my screen saver, my iPhone wallpaper, and print a hard copy for my night stand.

Later that day, I receive two emails from my new aunts Janet and Carol with a flurry of new details, anecdotes, enthusiasm, and love:

Hey Kimberly… I, too, want to join Rich in welcoming you into our family!

He was that little brother who loved playing tricks on the rest of us…

He loved to drop by for a few days, spoil [his nieces and nephews] with a lot of attention then take off for other adventures…

Your mother is beautiful—I can see why Chuck couldn't let her walk on by. I am so happy that you are the result!

When we were in high school he relentlessly dated all of my

friends (he was beautiful and easy to love). So when we got your letter…we weren't surprised AT ALL to find out about you!

It's probably better to digest us in small doses—together we are a swarm of family!

Thank you for being so courageous. I'm certain that we will all get a chance to meet and we look forward to that happy day.

Welcome Kimberly!

There it is again. *Welcome.*

Why are these strangers so trusting and warm? We don't even have a DNA test confirming *our* relation—only that Eric is my half-sibling. I didn't expect this. I wanted it, but had heard too many DNA test nightmares to get my hopes up. But their responses make more sense to me than my next breath. If the tables were turned, I would answer in kind. These humans respond to life the way I do—with enthusiasm, curiosity and a streak of impulsivity. I wander around the house with a stupid, disbelieving grin on my face for weeks, months.

But sharing the story with friends and coworkers is different. With each retelling, I grow more manic, more unsteady—my voice high, my hands shaking. I am strapped into a roller coaster that won't stop—overwhelming, exhilarating, terrifying all at once. The further I go, the further I slip outside myself. My body is a frayed electrical circuit, grounding wires ripped out, sparking, buzzing, untethered. I don't know how to do this.

Each time after recounting the story, I wish I hadn't. But I can't *not*; it flies out of me, trying to find a place to nest and rest. And that place is not me. With each syllable of his name—Charlie, Charles, Chuck—I lose another Newton of gravity.

Some friends have a hard time understanding my reaction. They are estranged from their fathers, forced to build identities without them. I take their words in and feel that familiar shame creep in—*Why am I grieving someone I never knew? I had a great dad, why do I need another? And why can't I find a foothold, a hand hold, an anything-hold to steady myself?*

Soon, I will be floating, swallowed up by space. My body will remind me of itself; it will whine, *what about me?*

CHAPTER 23

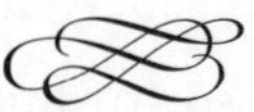

I TRAVEL for work in November and December and continue to vomit the story to anyone with ears—photo crews, Uber drivers, baristas, armrest-sharing airplane passengers. My inbox fills with communications—Rich, Carol and Janet—and also new cousins. And second cousins. I barely know my first cousins from Mom and Dad's bloodlines so this is an entirely new experience of family. My eldest cousin sends recipes that our grandma (grandma!) Isabelle loved to make (and Charlie loved to eat.) Others email cherished memories and photos. Janet shares two self-published collections of his poetry, Carol an elaborate genealogy tree that dates back to the 17th century. A file in my closet balloons with Charlie's old post-cards, photo prints, fliers, business cards, even rejection letters from publishers. This family holds tight to the ones they love.

One package from Rich contains a compilation of his favorite "Chuck tunes" burned onto a CD. I immediately copy it over to my music library.

All the tracks are written and sung by Charlie except one. Fellow Michigander and musician Neil Woodward, moved by Charlie's untimely death, wrote a lyrical ballad titled *Dark Mystery*. At the end of the tune, Neil weaves in a few stanzas from Charlie's *Whippoorwill*

—a short a cappella song recorded in rounds. Charlie's voice lilts and echoes the bird's sweet, lonesome call: *Gone to bed is the setting sun / night is coming and day is done / whippoorwill, whippoorwill has just begun…*

Though Neil never knew Charlie, his lyrics feel intimate, holding me in the somber tragedy of a life that "goes by too fast." His song helps me inch closer to feeling what I can't yet feel. I email Neil to thank him and he replies with a haunting story about the making of the song.

I wish you could have been in the studio when we flew Charlie's "Whippoorwill" into my recording. I truly cannot describe how spooked we were, as his presence in the room was so physical. Still gives me goosebumps when I hear it. I had not conceived of having his voice in there, I have no idea of how or when the concept occurred to me. Nevertheless, when we hit the record button, there he was, and now there he remains! Al, the engineer commented that Charles came in exactly as he was supposed to. I couldn't speak for quite a while, it seemed like it was out of our control. How could I write and play a completely different song, and wind up in the last twelve bars at the exact tempo and pitch as Charlie's 25 year old vinyl record? We sure weren't gonna mess with it, needless to say.

I fantasize, if Charlie mysteriously showed up during Neil's creation, maybe he'd come out and play with me too?

I am undeniably a product of Charlie's DNA—his physicality, his affinities, his nature. But I long to know the nurture of him. The part of our relationship that was never lived, yet somehow still unfolding.

So I do what I know how to do: I write. Not to answer him, but to reach for him. His words become a tether, a current I step into. I read his poetry—not to match it, but to listen. To hear his rhythms, his alliterations, his breath between the lines. To let his language settle in my bones and see if it stirs something dormant, something inherited, something already mine.

I don't have his training, but the act of writing—of shaping words into meaning—is my way of becoming his daughter. The eager-to-please child. The anxious, bun-headed dancer. The seeker longing for proof of a belonging that can never be spoken aloud.

His writing is the call; my writing is the response. A conversation between the living and the dead. A call across time. A message not etched in stone, but carried forward in breath, in ink, into the body of a life still unfolding.

NOVEMBER 30, 2014

Dear Charlie,

Is it possible to leave a part of yourself behind? You once asked this in a poem—did you already know the answer?

I've spent these past few months gathering pieces. A song on an old record. A close-up of your hands on a grainy TV screen. A crooked pinky. A family that never forgot you,. Your trail is scattered across time and space—in houses, in hearts, on hillsides, on stages, in words left behind.

But what takes your place? I do.

Not in the sense of filling your absence, but in continuing the movement—breathing new life into the parts you left behind. Your voice in my lungs. Your gaze behind my lens. Your story inside these pages.

No part is greater than the whole. No single remnant more meaningful than the others. But together—you, me, these echoes—we find our way.

CHAPTER 24

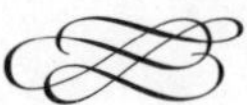

As my conversations with the Brauers continue and deepen, something shifts in Mom. At first, she holds back—perhaps out of propriety, or the lingering remnants of old shame—but as she watches the way they receive me, she begins to soften. Then, slowly, steps forward. Any last thread of her "Parson Larson" reserve unravels as she, too, is embraced with open arms.

This could have gone wrong in a thousand-and-one ways, but instead the Brauers lead with love.

My grandfather Carl Brauer's obituary reads: "His most lasting legacy is surely with his family. He and Isabelle lived very deliberately to create a close and loving family with bonds that have affected and included all the generations to this day." And though I never got to meet Carl or Isabelle, I'm humbled to be welcomed, truly welcomed, into their legacy.

I never fathomed a sequel to Mom's musing "*you belong to the mystery*," nor a mystery with real names, laughter and lineage. I feel sometimes as if Charlie, wearing a cloak of invisibility, is performing a magic trick on all of us. Am I the rabbit pulled from the hat? The Brauers lost a son, brother, uncle and cousin, they grieved the loss, adapted to life without him, and then three decades later, I show up. This kind of magic is not for the faint of heart—many would choose to shove the rabbit back in the hat, or claim she's not real. But I am real, as are my family. So the soft, innocent question of belonging sweeps us into each other's arms.

But a Dark Mystery still remains.

It's improbable that Charlie's fate was anything other than a tragic drowning. And I want to leave it at that. But when random anecdotes and details surface to suggest otherwise, my conviction wavers. And then fantasy gets the better of me and I entertain alternate realities where my biological dad returns—at a film premiere of his life story, a private message from 23andMe, in the comments of a serialized Substack memoir shared online.

Late December, Carol sends a package containing a photocopied entry from one of his journals. The actual diaries are boxed in their sister Janet's garage; she is poring through them slowly, gleaning insight into his hidden persona—the stuff we work out on our own or with a therapist and don't imagine someday, someone, might read them. But I get it. I read a few of Dad's journals after his death, hoping to find a phrase that would help me understand—what, I don't know. With no goodbye or closure, I'm glad I'm not the only one trying to make sense of the senseless.

I unfold the barely legible journal entry. I relate to his hastiness—emotions spilling onto paper have no pretense. There's no time to make it look good and urgency precedes craft. I am careless when I put thoughts on paper with pen in hand. I don't want to waste time constructing ideas, I just need black-ink validation. It takes time to decipher his words but I like that his messy script forces a slowdown.

I hold the first page up to the light. It's the premise for a serialized fiction column he's considering for *Sailing Magazine*:

A young man sells his car and drains his accounts to purchase a wooden sailboat, only to learn that the seller didn't own the boat, it had been stolen. He can't simply turn the boat over to the cops because he'd lose everything. And because he has no solid proof of purchase, with the boat now in his possession, he becomes the primary suspect.

[…]

He fails to clear himself and resorts to a fake drowning. A storm comes up, he abandons the boat at sea, making it look as if he had fallen overboard but really just disappears aboard another boat his confidant is piloting. The boat is found adrift and the young man (after an extensive search) is presumed drowned. His plan succeeds—the boat is returned to its rightful owner and the young man is clear by default. It's hard to prosecute a dead man. He is free to start anew.

I flip back to the first page for a date. Charlie wrote the story six months before he disappeared—in a sailing accident.

While going through Charlie's home after his disappearance, his siblings also discovered on a shelf, *How to Disappear Completely and Never Be Found.* This succinct guide for starting a new identity includes chapters on planning a disappearance, arranging for new identification, finding work, establishing credit, and pseudocide (creating the impression of one's own death).

My head spins. Like Schrödinger's cat, Charlie is trapped in quantum possibility. He is both alive *and* dead—our grief boxed in eternal uncertainty.

I look back through emails with the Brauers. Rarely do they write "died" or "deceased." Instead, they use words like "vanished," "disappeared," and "went missing." When a body is never recovered, it makes sense to use these words. But do they actually question his death? What in his character would make pseudocide even the remotest of possibilities? When they share anecdotes and describe Charlie as "spontaneous" and "mischievous," just how mischievous? Arriving at family gatherings unannounced, charming the pants off nieces and nephews and then disappearing without notice for months at a time is odd, but not pathologically odd. The desire for a clean slate, a fresh start and a brand new day can sometimes be tempting, especially when up against a wall. But a solid, loving family renders this unthinkable or the executioner, unhinged.

I resolve: shipwrecked with finitude at the bottom of Lake Michigan.

And still: I'll keep reading comments and private DMs with bated breath.

CHAPTER 25

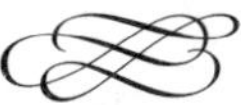

OVER THE LAST NINE YEARS, I've sporadically researched community-based housing options for adults with intellectual disability. I want to believe Syd's future is bright—filled with peers, agency and dignity—but both state and private establishments are often lacking or inaccessible, so families become full-time caregivers. And Syd, while abundantly sunny, is full time—physically, mentally, emotionally. This scenario haunts me and its implication on our lives. And muffled under the fear, a mountain of guilt and shame for feeling the way I do. Many of our vetted homes have eight to ten-year wait lists. Syd's half-sister Mac (a few years younger and wise beyond years) has expressed interest in caregiving someday and we hold onto that as a possibility, but she's still in high school. We also explore turning Dave's four-bedroom rental into a home with staffed aides and a few additional residents.

Possibilities are discussed but never land. We limp along with a half-baked strategy impinged by unprocessed trauma and immobilizing terror—the history of care for persons with intellectual disability is fraught with stigma, mistreatment and neglect.

During the holidays, Dave receives a message from an unexpected source—a warning of upheaval ahead. A vague but foreboding note that, at first, we brush off. But within weeks, the situation unravels, and reality crashes down. The fragile balance we've relied on for years is suddenly gone. Syd's weekday care, already tenuous, collapses overnight. For years, she's been shuttled between homes, caregivers, and schedules that keep changing, an arrangement that was never ideal but one we convinced ourselves could hold until something better came along. We knew a more permanent solution was needed—we just thought we had more time to find it.

Now, time is up. A future we thought we were inching toward is suddenly here, and we are wildly unprepared. The conversations, the ideas, the contingency plans we batted around for years are no longer theoretical. There is no more waiting for the "right" solution to present itself. The decision has been made for us.

Underneath a frozen tundra of denial, molten panic inflames my blood.

And now Dave—my rock, my foundation, the roots that pull me back to earth—is yanked from shore. spinning in the chaos of his own worst nightmare-come-true. I want to be his lifeline, but there's nothing solid to grab ahold—I'm already unmoored. We flail together, reaching arms out to one another for salvation, but the storm is too great.

The drowning can't save the drowning.

As the unknown erodes us from within, we grasp for the known. Meals still need to be prepared, clients still need our time, plans still need to be made. We take steps forward, however inconsequential, to ground ourselves in the imminent tempest, and I grasp for any branch of hope, goodness or solidarity I can find.

After Christmas, I email Carol, Janet and Rich and impulsively suggest we meet in person in the spring. Less than two hours later all three reply with a reverberating *Yes*.

My body makes no distinction between fear and excitement. Disney or doom, cells respond all the same. I lose words, my core trembles, senses question, sleep evades. This is nothing new. Even in my youth, Dad would meet my nighttime anxiety with a reassuring hand on back and teach box breathing. I was never successful at smoothing the energy that blazed through me. But eventually, nerves would reset and a semblance of calm returned. But now I can't find my reset button. I lay in bed and imagine Dad massaging my feet, drawing energy downwards, but it doesn't work. I try my other method; I ask Dave to lay his entire body's length on top of me, shoving me into gravity. I am loose silt compressing under the heavy, certain earth of his body. My cells listen and try to remember. But they slip, I slide, fear floods.

What have I done?

* * *

In early January, I travel to Mexico for a catalog job, arriving a day early to settle in, take a walk on the beach, and rest before the long, hot days ahead. The next six days will be a blur—early call times, relentless sun, little time to unwind.

My friend and crew member Destiny also arrives a day early, so we meet for lunch on an upstairs patio. Over two bowls of tortilla soup, she viscerally recounts one of the scariest days of her life. Just four months ago, this healthy, bright, twenty-six-year-old beauty had a stroke. I listen, breath halted in my chest, as she describes the harrowing experience of a body's command center undone.

My cells are listening too. They hear panic, and can't distinguish it from their own.

I go green. I recognize this sensation—I have blacked-out easily a dozen times as an adult—due to that "strong vasovagal response." But while sitting down? Usually it's triggered by chronic low blood pressure or diabolical menstrual cramps. I stand up instinctively, reaching for a bench a few paces away. Not a good idea. My vision closes in and I'm out, face-planting on the hard concrete.

When I return to consciousness, I hear Destiny calling for help. My leggings are wet with urine and my nose bloody. When staff and crew members surround, I casually brush it off. "I pass out a lot." "Maybe I was dehydrated." "Maybe I was hungry." But when I return to the privacy and safety of my room, I tremble with worry. I can't for the life of me figure out why this happened. Armed with food and electrolytes everywhere I go, I know for certain I wasn't dehydrated. Or hungry.

I call Eric. I need to feel something—someone—solid.

He answers the phone. I adore my brother's voice. It is sap. It is thick, dark molasses for my raw nerves. Eric is enveloping, unwavering reassurance. "Aw sis. You're strong. You're going to be fine. Take it easy. Eat a banana, just in case." Two bananas later, I take a nap, join the crew for dinner and work the next six days. Other than a lingering angst about my unexplainable blackout, I feel completely normal. And thanks to Destiny's magic make-up, careful positioning of my face to hide the swelling, and Photoshop, I look normal too.

But when I return to Portland for another week of catalog work, my body sounds an alarm again. *What about me! Listen to me!*

Driving to the photo studio—a route I've traveled countless times—the road suddenly undulates and flips. My stomach follows suit. I inhale, focus, steady hands on wheel, exhale. But inside, it's a gymnasium—vaulting, spinning, unstable. I ease onto the shoulder, gripping reality as it wobbles beneath me. *What the hell is going on?* I try to breathe deeply. I tell myself, *I'm fine. I'm fine. I'm fine. I think I can, I think I can, I think I can.* I sit. Wait. Turn on NPR to distract escalating nerves. Eventually the tumbling routine settles, and I get back on the highway and drive to work. The car's dash reads normal but my body's check engine light is flashing dangerously red.

As my 40th birthday approaches, I spend days filming and editing a series of video journals for a local non-profit. When I stand up from late night editing sessions, my chest fills with ice, hypothermic jitters rattle my ribs. I take scalding baths to warm up but the heat can't penetrate the deep freeze settling in.

My birthday comes and goes without much fanfare. Eye-stabbing headaches settle in, and anxiety's inevitable twin—depression—moves closer. *Hi, Dad.* Dave plans a surprise birthday visit from family, but it falls through last minute. Only Eric, on a whim, still makes it. Our time together is brief but his effort is a lifeline. My sense of identity and how it fits into my family, my future with Dave, is unraveling. Birthday tacos and tequila make my head spin more than usual. I stay in bed after Eric leaves, numb catatonia the last refuge for nerves undone.

CHAPTER 26

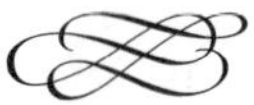

The Madison Historical Society houses twenty-five cans of film from Charlie's TV show *Long Ago is All Around*. I arrange to arrive a day early to my next gig in Wisconsin and binge-watch the footage —I've never been so eager to hang at a library all day. In an email to Rich, I mention my plans and he replies with one of his own:

"Guess what? My daughter Gretchen (Greta) who works in Chicago at a fancy ass bike shop is going to be in Madison next week from Sunday to Wednesday. Apparently there's a bike show or something there. I just talked to her and told her of your plans. She'd love to connect with her newfound cousin. She's 31. You'll love her. I told her not to pick her nose in front of you since she'll be the first Brauer you'll meet. She said that she would behave herself. I don't know if this will work with your schedule, but I hope it does. P.S. Save the trip to the library. I have copies of those episodes from his TV series. Perhaps for a plate of cookies, I'll get you a DVD sometime."

Gulp. I could bail. I could tell a white lie and say the photo shoot was canceled. I could change the dates. My mind spins with a string of escape plans. Now that it's real, I don't know if I'm ready. I thought I was, but my body disagrees. I read Rich's email again; he is so casual, so non-threatening. He makes this inaugural meet-up seem normal and easy, like two old friends grabbing a beer.

I'm on a treadmill and I can't get off. From the moment I first received the DNA results, a momentum far outside my control has been in charge. I cycle from manically excited to totally wiped out two to three times a day. The treadmill keeps running but my body trips over itself trying to keep up.

I say yes—partially because I don't want to disappoint and appear like the high-strung ball of nerves that I am, and partially because I r*eally, really do* want to meet my newfound family. And now, there's no denying it—Greta has officially appeared in my DNA Relatives on 23andMe: first cousin. The digital breadcrumb trail has led to something real, something irrefutable. I want to get through this everything-is-scary-and-new phase and the only way to do it is to dive in. Friends say I've been "brave" these last six months. I don't feel brave at all. Communicating behind screens is one thing but meeting a family member in the flesh makes me want to tear up the script and hide.

A few short hours after I arrive in Madison, Greta and I will meet. *In person.* I check into my room, unsure of where or how to sit on the hotel bed. I watch myself play-act "chill"—flipping through channels, not checking the time every five minutes, not noticing my shaking hands, not fooling anyone. I try a few nervous system hacks but they only red alert my brain even more—*You're watching your breath…are we in danger? You're in child's pose…are we not safe?*—so I let them go. I'm keen to meet this bright, young woman and learn about her life, her family. Our family. If I can stay focused on Greta, maybe I won't leave the earth's atmosphere.

When the sun sets, I drive to the city center and park a block from the bar, ignoring the spot out front. I need some time to put sneaker on pavement. A walk along one city block isn't enough to integrate past, present and my imminent future but it at least paves the way.

I am intentionally early. Instead of scanning the room as I enter, I walk straight to the bar and order a shot of tequila, poured into a glass for sipping. I would love to order two doubles and down the first before Greta arrives, but I can't trust it to help. Lately, it only seems to sharpen the edge rather than dull it. Instead, I wait, eyes fixed on the door. *The next time it opens, it's going to be her—my cousin. She's going to be early too.*

The bartender thumps down a lowball glass and my heart replies with a racing thrum, just as a stunning, rosy-cheeked young woman bounds through the doors, catches my eye, and before I can say "OH MY GOD" she's in my arms.

Her embrace—the first true warm day of spring. Tentative limbs abandon apprehension and lean in.

I'd be happiest simply sitting next to Greta in silence, shoulder-to-shoulder, melting in her warmth. But of course, that's not what strangers—or perhaps even cousins— do.

While she talks, I steal into her eyes, study her face, and I see, *I feel,* myself. Her bone structure, skin tone, mouth, but even more, her essence. Cells light up, one-by-one, a galaxy of dying stars reignited by a mirrored dimension of itself. I lean into the gestalt of our resonance. And though she was born after Charlie's disappearance, she speaks as if he never disappeared.

This family never let Charlie go. No wonder I'm so welcome. In a strange way, through me, they are getting their long-lost tribe member back. *I hope I don't disappoint.*

Early into the evening Rich can't bear to be out of the conversation. He phones Greta. She picks up and says, "Yup, she's right here! Yup, it's amazing! Ok, hang on." *Hang on? Uh oh.* I think I'm about to connect with Brauer #2. It's becoming uncomfortably clear how easy it is to hide behind texts and emails. There is time to reflect and edit, there is a generous cushion of space surrounding each correspondence. Now, I'm in real time with real voices, real flesh and the real possibility of completely losing my shit.

Greta smiles wide encouragement and hands me the phone, "Take it into the bathroom so you can hear better." I laugh, curse and comply. Before I can even lock the restroom door I hear a jolly, "Kimberly! Welcome to the family!" Here he is. My dad's brother. My uncle. His familiar midwestern accent and warm enthusiasm are a balm for frayed nerves, reminding cells of their origin. Both Greta and Rich radiate an unquestioning love that says, *You're here to stay*. The door of my heart swings open wide.

Though exhausted, I lay wide awake all night long, replaying moments, details—a film student's cheesy montage worms into my brain. I should've had a second tequila, a third. My nerves can't come down from all the excitement. Around 6:00am I finally get an hour of escape but cortisol sounds her 7:00am alarm and I'm awake for the day. So I hit the road. I need to be on location by evening, so I take the day to mirror-neuron the unwinding rural roads. The flat, late-winter landscape, frozen lakes, the sleeping fields—these scenes quiet me. There's also a house near the Mississippi River border I want to visit, though I'm sure it's inhabited. I route my GPS to Ferryville, a western Wisconsin border town (if a bar and a church make it so) where Charlie spent the last three years of his life, in a home built with his own two hands.

I listen to NPR as I drive. Just when I turn into the Ferryville township, Writer's Almanac guest, Jeffery Harrison, reads his poem, "A Drink of Water":

When my nineteen-year-old son turns on the kitchen tap
and leans down over the sink and tilts his head sideways
to drink directly from the stream of cool water,
I think of my older brother, now almost ten years gone,
who used to do the same thing at that age;
and when he lifts his head back up and, satisfied,
wipes the water dripping from his cheek
with his shirtsleeve, it's the same casual gesture
my brother used to make; and I don't tell him
to use a glass, the way our father told my brother,
because I like remembering my brother
when he was young, decades before anything
went wrong, and I like the way my son
becomes a little more my brother for a moment
through this small habit born of a simple need,
which, natural and unprompted, ties them together
across the bounds of death, and across time …
as if the clear stream flowed between two worlds
and entered this one through the kitchen faucet,
my son and brother drinking the same water.

My car slows as I turn right onto a gravel road, the same road

Charlie drove every day to and from his home, *this small habit born of a simple need / which, natural and unprompted, ties them together / across the bounds of death, and across time…* and I can't help but wonder, what small habit born of simple need do I have that ties me across the bounds of death to Charlie?

I grab my phone from the passenger seat and dial Rich's phone number. I do it quickly, not giving my mind enough time to comprehend the magnitude of the act. The only way to accomplish this simple task is to do it, but my stomach leaps into my throat anyway. I want to sound casual so I lead with an enthusiasm as true as the gnarled knot in my stomach. He's at his film studio when he picks up.

"Well hey there Kimberly! How the heck are you? Are you on Rush Creek Road?"

Rich hasn't been to his brother's home in a long time, but he remembers the gravel road well enough and offers to be my GPS. The road winds into a deep valley. The hills on either side are crowded with bare trees. March is too risky for vulnerable, spring buds. I go in and out of cell reception so when I find a property that looks like a possibility, I snap a shot with my phone and then drive back out to the main road to send to Rich. I do this three or four times, pausing in front of each prospective house to imagine Charlie on the stoop, Ranger at his feet. *Is this the one? Did he plant that tree? Did he have coffee on that porch?* My first solid connection with Uncle Rich (other than the brief bathroom phone call) is a playful scavenger hunt, not a sit-down "Who are you?" and "What is the meaning of life?" Having grown up with much of the latter, I'm all in.

Rich guides, "Keep looking for a third floor writer's nook. It will be the tell-tale sign you've found Chuck's house. There may be an outhouse nearby and a small-ish creek also runs through the property." *An outhouse? What century did Charlie live in?* I stop my car a half-dozen times to feel the breeze on my face. Even though I haven't found his property yet, I inhale the air he breathed. I listen, Charlie's long-lost days songbird into me.

Eventually, way further into the valley than Rich expected, I come upon a freshly painted, two-story house (and a tiny, third story nook!) with a small, bubbling creek cutting through the yard. The trees near the house are medium size, about what I'd expect if Charlie planted them thirty years earlier. My mind plants him into the empty front porch—a lanky, ash-blonde man sits with an open journal, paused. A coonhound rests at his feet and thumps his tail. Inside, a table is set for two, staged exactly the way his siblings found it the day he sailed across Lake Michigan and never returned. Charlie lived alone, so is this setting a ritual act of comfort or hope?

It looks like no one is home so I pull my car to the side of the dirt road and cautiously trespass. Winter thaws as the early afternoon sun builds confidence. Birds chatter about and the creek replies. I take a few audio recordings on my phone. I want to return to these sounds, eyes closed, body transported. I squat down beside the creek, mud pushing up alongside the soles of my sneakers, and listen *as if the clear stream flowed between two worlds / and entered this one;* this was Charlie's happy place, and it would've also been mine.

For a moment, we can be here, alone, together.

Our shared solitude dulls anxious shards in my belly. We lie in the grass, our thoughts unfurling new possibilities. We listen to trees while I record their knowledge in my own, timid and unformed roots.

* * *

I work for two days with an all-female crew and share the paternity story over dinner—the women's generous warmth an invitation I can't resist. I laugh. I smile. I am genuinely enthusiastic. The engaged storyteller in me is on a roll, but as usual, my needle wavers. Another part of me prays I stop sharing and slow down the hands of time. She wants to integrate too but needs it *her* way—quiet, attuned, glacial. Like undiscovered life in the great ocean depths, she shies from the light of the world, nurtured instead by the chthonic, steady pulse of patient darkness.

After the shoot I drive to Madison for an evening flight home, but the plane is overbooked and I trade my seat for a $500 voucher and a morning flight. I surrender to a night of nothingness, lying on my hotel bed as dusk unspools herself from the bedding, the marred laminate table, the curtains, me. Even gloaming is too much light when the mind is on fire. Darkness is food. Silence, medicine. Eventually grounded enough to fulfill a simple, basic need, I decide: eat dinner, drink a glass of wine, people-watch other dramas. Tonight, mine is on pause.

But when I take a seat at the hotel bar, the floor flips up.

Again? What now, body?

I walk as calmly as possible to the restroom, steadying my gaze on the path as it liquifies beneath my feet. *It's not safe here. I'm not safe here.* Behind a locked door, I slide down to the concrete floor and press my back into the wall. It yields to my weight and fear pushes it over.

I sit for too long, begging to feel sound—my own company, this body, no kind companion.

CHAPTER 27

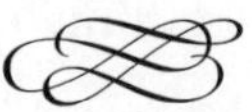

Charlie's life ended on eighteen-foot Lake Michigan swells. And now, I join him.

By early April, occasional dizzy spells churn into an unremitting tempest. Unlike ocean swells and their corduroy predictability, our inland waves aren't driven by tides, refuse directionality and change on a dime. Our waves threaten disaster. Our waves take life.

Dave is concerned but for the most part, my symptoms are invisible. He doesn't share my new life at sea. He can't envision the volatile shifts—from giant swells to choppy waters—a neurological squall of misinterpreted signaling. He can't see the sidewalk liquify under my step as we walk around the block to "shake it off." But he does see a shrinking me, an unrecognizable me—a once-daring tomboy, now-overly cautious, timid and disoriented by slight changes in my environment. He's as scared and desperate as I am, especially as the sudden demands of becoming Syd's full-time guardian parallel my descent.

My primary care doctor shrugs and refers me to an ENT. She's convinced *it'll pass* and I'm a good patient, so I nod, feign chipper, and agree. Nothing can last forever. I wrestle my way through once-effortless tasks—brushing my teeth while standing at the mirror? Clown house. Conversing? I can't focus on you. Sleeping? Forget about it. My stomach curls itself into cowering prey under the bewildered stares of clients, grocery clerks, ER docs, family. I bail on commitments. My phone pinging or a simple knock on the door sends me into rib-prickling panic.

Before heading to Orcas Island on another catalog gig, I ask the producer if any doctors or acupuncturists or shamans or healers or witchdoctors or miracle workers or exorcists on the island can heal me. I am desperate. If nothing else, at least I can book a few appointments—a place to lie down at the end of the work day and feel safe, and not alone with the sensations. I make three appointments with a Native American shaman/acupuncturist; if necessary, I will spend my entire week's pay to get through each day. But instead of getting better, the sensations foment and intensify. Electric shocks spark my torso. Sharp pain digs at the base of my skull. My tongue goes numb. When on my back, I'm upside down. When standing, a rude force yanks me starboard and under. *Take me, I'm already under.*

The shaman suggests: "Kundalini experience?"

I reject: *Shove the snake back in the basket for another lifetime. I can't do this.*

The last night on Orcas I pull myself together and join the crew for a wrap dinner. My sunniness isn't fooling anyone, especially myself, but going through the motions helps me believe the sensations will disappear as spontaneously as their arrival. But the restaurant is deafening, every voice in the room punches with equal intensity and volume. Silver on ceramic, a pitchfork into eardrum. The tea lights carve mean angles into my eyes. I order steak frites—something grounding. But I can't hold it together anymore; my brain is sounding so many alarm bells I think it might explode. I steal away, unsure if I'm walking in a straight line, and then *at last* out of sight, I gasp for air.

Destiny is here with me on this trip, too. She sees me, clocking the shift in my body, and follows. She knows everything—makeup artists just do. Spending hours together on a job, often with no more than six inches between faces, gut-busting laughter and heart-wrenching vulnerability become part of the shared territory. With pencils and brushes animating our stories, I've known more intimacy with makeup artists than with some exes.

Destiny grabs me into her arms and we cry. Her presence is an anchor, but I'm already slipping, disappearing into the unlit night sky. It's much safer up there. After a long, unsteady silence, she pulls back, wipes my face, and throws a steady arm around my waist, guiding me back to my room.

A few minutes later, she returns with a dinner tray. "Do you want company?"

I want to say yes. I want someone to hold me down to the ground, to press me into the earth with weight. To tell me I'm safe—and for once, I want to believe them. But I don't feel safe anywhere, least of all in this body. I want to disappear, to dissociate, and I can't with someone near.

"I think I just need to eat dinner and crash, I'll be better in the morning."

She hesitates, hearing what I don't say. "Okay, my ringer is on loud if you need me."

The door closes, swallowing the last sliver of hallway. I lie on my back staring at nothing as sensory input fractures distorts, severing me into nothing. I look down at a woman who appears normal, but inside—a hellscape.

Shock waves tear through her torso, she looks around the room, unable to distinguish floor from ceiling, gravity pulls from all four directions at once, she weighs five hundred pounds, then a feather. Voices in the hall blade into her chest, she's hungry but can't eat riding bareback in a bouncy castle at sea. Hot tingling, painful tingling everywhere. her dinner tray is on the floor next to the bed and every half-hour, she rolls off the mattress—hands, knees, hips, full recline— shoveling spoonfuls into her mouth. Prayers delivered on meat and potatoes, she sips water, certain it's been laced with LSD. The hotel carpet is a soft friend, she needs a soft friend, she presses her cheek into poly-fiber weave, shrinking her awareness down to each scratchy nub. A distraction from existence. but when an angry rumbling at the base of her skull rises—louder, deafening, demanding incarnation—

I return to my body and it starts all over again.

I scream silently.

* * *

I return home and more shoulder shrugs unravel hope. The ENT writes a referral to a neurologist. The bike incident last year misleads and prolongs a diagnosis—there are insurance codes for traumatic brain injury and post-concussion syndrome, none for an unraveling identity and losing one's shit. So with four more months of desperate waiting on my calendar, I move forward with life, hanging on to what little threads of it I have left.

In early May, I head back to the airport for another short gig in Wisconsin. I sit in the ~~gate area~~ bouncy castle as a troop of sugar-jacked monkeys tumble around me. I now live 24/7 on a strange planet and I can't adapt. My body's new homeostasis—terror.

I watch everyone board the plane but I remain in my seat. *I think I can, I think I can. Get on that plane, Kim.* First class boards. Families and special needs. A little girl claws at her dad's leg until he picks her up. *I think I can, I think I can.* Section A, B, C, then D. The gate is full of traveler buzz and then empty. *I think I can, I think I can.* I hear the flight attendant call my name. Once, twice, three times. I don't budge while tears flood my eyes.

I can't.

The gate closes.

I freeze in my seat. Life literally flies by at airports—the full catastrophe of love, dreams, loss and disappointment are held within every terminal and then lifted and landed by wings. My insignificant nightmare is dulled by the busyness and I need it this way. I step outside it all. The woman I used to be is on that plane, headed to a silly job to collect a silly paycheck and then she will continue her silly existence. This other woman, the one whose sitz bones are glued into a chair at Gate 36 can't see the future. She can't even figure out what the next fifteen minutes look like. So she doesn't do anything at all. Travelers rush to their gates and she recognizes the pace. Her life changed too fast but now she can't stop it.

She needs uneventful. She needs boredom. No new aunts and uncles to meet. No new cousins. No new dad.

I rewind events and think about my choices. I could have said no to meeting the Brauers this year. I could've waited. Should've? But that would've delayed the inevitable. I could have never written the letter, but then a part of me would always be in hiding. I could've never taken the DNA test but then the mystery wins. I could've never typed "Charlie Brauer musician Wisconsin" into the search bar, but how many things do we Google every day, not expecting it to change the course of our lives?

I don't know how long I sit at the gate. Minutes? Hours? Eventually reason breaks through my trance. I have to call my agent, tell her I'm not on the plane. I have to tell her what's happening to me. But I don't *know* what's happening to me. Admitting this to her, giving voice to my circumstances, makes it more real. I can no longer fake my way through this with a smile. Now my agency knows. Soon, all my clients will know. Soon, my income will disappear.

And now I have to call Dave. I need a ride home.

I dial. It rings. I picture him at home, maybe pouring a drink, maybe standing in the kitchen, his body already relaxing into early evening. The normalcy of that image is unbearable.

"Hello?" He answers, clipped. He already knows something's wrong. I was supposed to be in the air.

"Dave? I—" My breath hitches. "I'm still at the airport. I didn't miss my flight. I mean, I did. I mean, I didn't get on the plane."

Silence. A pause thick with calculation. His brain mapping my words trying to make sense of them. "What?"

"I just—" My chest tightens. "I couldn't. Something happened. I—I don't know what happened."

Another pause. And then simply:

"I'm on my way."

No questions, no reassurances, just action. Just motion.

Dave's trauma response is also of the popsicle variety. Occasionally our respective ice pops melt a little and we have an outburst of emotion, but when Dave's already stressed, my neediness plummets the mercury in his blood. I've learned there's a right time to let loose or I'll re-traumatize myself, crying for help with no one to rescue. Underneath the freeze, Dave is terrified as he watches his independent, capable, optimistic-to-a-fault partner unravel. Now he has two adult dependents, and for the first time, that encumbrance is breaking him.

So for now, we think, as long as we keep moving, check boxes, continue our momentum, the hot catastrophe in our hearts will be protected by glacial sheets of frost.

And we do; we keep moving. We try.

* * *

We'd booked our upcoming trip to Michigan—the much-anticipated meeting with the Brauers— right around the time Syd's caregiving situation began to unravel. Maybe we didn't fully trust how bad things would get, or maybe we simply couldn't fathom it, so we moved ahead, believing stability would hold. But now, with the trip just two weeks away, that trust feels naïve. The ground beneath us has buckled, but we've arranged for caregivers in shifts, 24/7, at Dave's rental. But as we drive home in silence, I start canceling everything in my head. There's no way I'm ready to meet my biological family. They are strangers and I'm a mess. But I can't cancel. I won't. This family, my family—we are only a few calls and emails young. We need time together to render time inconsequential.

But as the date of our departure looms, I only get worse.

On May 17th, the night before our flight and wan with shame and embarrassment, I send off a sunny, yet apologetic forewarning.

Dear Carol, Janet and Rich,

I'm so looking forward to spending time with you this week. I have been putting something off—hoping for a miracle and am still holding out for one—but it's better I fill you in now than after we arrive.

I've been experiencing some crazy debilitating dizziness this past month and have been in and out of doctor visits trying to get to the bottom of it. I feel so embarrassed and scared to share this totally-out-of-sorts me with all of you. I want nothing more than to be strong and share my fullest heart with you and not worry about this. These symptoms just really have a hold of me in a way I've never experienced.

We fly out tomorrow, arriving in Traverse City later in the day. My mantra tonight and tomorrow is that WE WILL GET ON THAT PLANE. Making this trip is so very important to me and it may even be healing on some deeper level. Who knows. I do wish I didn't have to send this email at all, arriving tomorrow in full spirits so we get on with living and loving.

I press send, praying the next ice age descends overnight and all flights are canceled indefinitely.

At 6:55am on May 18th, Dave and I board our plane, my heart's flight fueled with their reassurance:

We love you. Even if you're only up for a hug, that's fine with us. We just want you to be well. We're all happy to be here together so no pressure on when you are able to connect. It doesn't have to be for long. And did we mention that we love you?

* * *

Dave and I arrive in Michigan midday, his steady hand mending mine since liftoff. We stock up on groceries en route to our rental; the grocery cart a cherished walker as I navigate the animated aisles —boxes of cereal and soup cans a kaleidoscopic hell. I'm a collision of sensations and emotions so the only option is to go with it. During the one-hour drive to our cabin, I look out the window and enjoy temporary relief from symptoms—as long as I'm in passive motion, the 24/7 rocking, bobbing, and swaying disappear. And not just a little— completely. But as soon as the car stops, even if for just a moment, sensations return full force and clobber. I learn with time to do a slow, 2 mph creep at stoplights so the tsunami of motion doesn't hit while obeying traffic signals.

Our rental is on Crystal Lake, Michigan's inland-Mediterranean; the Brauer family cottage is twenty minutes down shore near the sleepy town of Beulah. Carol and Janet have already arrived, enjoying their sisterly bond and buzzing with anticipation. I buzz too, but like a downed line, arcing and sparking with anxiety.

My body needs cycles and seasons to metabolize, traveling not at the speed of thought, but at the speed of inhale—sunrise—exhale—sunset. Winter—spring—summer—fall. My organs and humors take time to integrate and digest new, foreign nutrients. They understand the natural necessity of death and rebirth. But my ego doesn't trust this pace, she's scared to unravel into uncertain chaos. I go to bed, but I do not sleep. Electricity courses through my ribs, someone's ribs—this body is no longer mine. Someone's ears listen to water lapping ashore. Someone's brain thinks she's at sea, that waves underneath a mattress are normal. Time is slow and thoughts are both intrusive and out of reach. *This can't go on, why are you so bent out of shape? No one wants to see you like this, no one will love you like this, you're not safe, you're not safe, you're not safe.*

We rest our first day. Rest—less an actual reset as much as avoiding variables of unpredictability. When horizontal—the bed bouncing up and down—I pray, I visualize, I mental acupuncture myself. When standing, I pretend Dad or God or a friendly ghost is slow dance rocking me.

Late afternoon, in search of temporary relief, we drive around the lake to visit Charlie's memorial bench. Like a blissed out dog, I hang my head out the window—unfailingly calm and still when in motion. I cast myself in an endless roadtrip. When we reach Charlie's bench in the quiet harbor town of Frankfurt, we park the car and the waves return.

The bench is flanked by two, healthy, red maples. I want to be flanked by two red maples, rooting me. I sit on it and look out at the quiet harbor scene and imagine my biological father setting sail for the last time.

The plaque on the bench reads:

Charles Phillip Brauer

1949–1985

Journeyed from this port, September 23rd, 1985 bound for Sturgeon Bay. His years of sailing experience were no match for the deadly Lake Michigan storm. These trees and bench are placed as a memorial to Charles honoring his relationship with nature and its powerful beauty. He was loved and will be missed. "Now rest beneath blue waters—let praise to thy creator rise."—Brauer family—1986

The ground undulates as I read the dedication, imagining my biological father's own exit from solid ground. He never reached land again.

Will I?

The next morning Carol and Janet check in. They are happy to head our direction today—*just a simple drive along the lake shore to meet your deceased brother's daughter for the first time!* Are they having nervous breakdowns, too?

The doorbell rings and I answer. I am visibly shaking and sweating but I've prepared them. "I'm a mess, I'm not myself." Now all I can do is be exactly that—myself.

We embrace. My damp armpits staining the imagined perfect moment long ago abandoned. Dave politely hugs them and then steps back to observe and hold the space. He welcomes this distraction from life's heaviness—from Syd's struggles, from his, from mine. Today feels light, joyful even—and so very surreal. Any awkwardness thaws away as we curl up on the sofa and share stories. Carol and Janet both sit like I do—feet tucked under our butts, leaning heavily to one side—our shared body language, uncanny. But more than physical similarities, I feel a vibrational match—from dissonance to consonance, a chord progression is brought home. All the invisible stuff that makes up a self—how one senses a room, the way thought travels through flesh, how memory lives and dies, and the ineffable summation of presence—this spiritual harmonic is louder than anything I comprehend through five senses.

Rich joins us the next day for a drive around Benzie county—a stomping ground for Brauer generations. He grabs me into a giant bear hug when we meet, then takes Dave into his arms with equal affection. I felt this same joy and ease over the phone, but in person, I regress into preverbal necessity. The longing for *Dad* floods me. I feel five again. I want to curl up in his arms and stay forever.

We pile into a decades-loved Suburban. Carol's husband Harry chauffeurs while Rich plays tour guide in the passenger seat. In the back, Carol and Janet nestle on either side of me; Dave a comfortable bookend to the chorus line of estrogen. When he isn't holding or squeezing my hand, he photographs our grafting tree.

Benzie county a has been a family vacation stomping ground

for generations. Charlie had bought a home in the area so when the herds of family gathered for July 4th festivities, annual sauerkraut cook-offs and winter sports on the lake, he had a solitary escape. We drive by the humble, two-story house while Rich storyboards scenes:

"Ranger dragged a squirrel out of that tree and maimed it. Never one to waste anything, Chuck grilled it."

"On these sharp curves in the road, cherry trucks would lose some harvest. Chuck round up the fugitives and made his signature Road Kill Cherry Pie."

"Convinced television was rotting the human brain, Chuck took a shotgun to his right there."

Rich's stories are endless—it's easy to see why he got into filmmaking—every tree, curb, shack and bend in the road reanimates his big brother into 24 frames per second. There's Charlie—roguish, self-reliant, a lover of nature and the untamed. He welcomed surprise, he didn't like being tied down, and he preferred the open road to a mortgage. He used his charisma and charm to keep family and friends close, but not too close. The tales are mostly funny, lighthearted and well-rehearsed, as if they've been told around campfires, passed down through generations, eventually becoming the stuff of legends. And when you die young, legendary status is inevitable.

Our last day in Michigan, we reunite at the family cottage—its own immortal fame rivaling Charlie's. Isabelle and Carl, my grandparents, believed family always came first, and reinforced this value by creating a home base for frequent family gatherings. The tiny, twelve-hundred square foot cabin is so storied I can almost hear its own beating, knotty pine heart. I enter—the space around me familiar but distant, aching like a phantom limb.

Two to three dozen family members assemble at the cottage every July, with Carl's sisters' families just a few doors down. Bunk beds, a kitchen the size of a small pontoon, chairs pushed up against every free wall—even though there are only seven of us now, I can hear the quilt of voices, the laughing children, the wet, bare feet pounding up and down narrow staircase, the sweet melody of reunion as Isabelle and Carl's greatest wish is fulfilled. Their ghosts smile in every worn upholstery fiber, water glass ring and speck of dust.

I could walk around the interior perimeter in a minute or less, but the floor-to-ceiling family relics demand a museum pace—family portraits, framed poetry, hand-carved sculptures, illustrations, paintings, crayon-ings, a photo of Charlie sailing Fogbow, framed newspaper articles from the 60's and 70's on Charlie's budding music career, a painted-portrait of Charlie…

My deceased biological father is EVERYWHERE.

A cow hide hangs above a well-loved sofa, inscribed with generations of names. A hot tool hangs beside it. Every blood relative and spouse is branded into the great beast—a supple family tree with limbs unbound by direction, unlimited by reach. Dave and I scan and scan until we find Charlie's name. *There it is!* in his own handwriting, scribed no less than thirty-five years ago. I touch it, pressing my fingers into the mark, trying to wrinkle time—his hand and mine momentarily one.

And then, Rich hands me the tool.

Below Charlie's signature, I burn my own, fire on flesh, alchemical forever. This family relic is no erase board; belonging here is unending. And then they pass the torch to Dave, a gesture more enduring than our unmarried status. I lean into his warm body as he extends his arm into our unquestioned future.

To say the Brauers know how to make a person feel welcome is the understatement of a lifetime.

I wobble and sway through it all, desperately wanting to take in the fullness of experience. But, I drift through our first minutes and hours and days together, catching only glimpses of the tender details as they pass. There is laughter and lots of it. There are stories, more than I can remember. There are twinkling, teary eyes. Chocolate bars. Wind-whipped hair and nostalgia-whipped hearts. But what isn't present in focus, I make up for with infinite gratitude. This radiant clan extends to me an unwavering invitation into their lives. And they into mine. It is here, I am absolutely certain, that we meet.

When it's time to say goodbye I am relieved. I need to get horizontal, close my eyes and shut out the world. I've never been one to do the movie goodbye, no craning my head 180 degrees, waving until loved ones dissolve into the horizon. But here I am:

The frame widens: faces I've already memorized, sparkling eyes, generous smiles. Then the family picnic table, the little yellow house, the one next to it, the shared driveway. Crystal Lake peeks out from behind the neighborhood, winking in sunset glitter.

Windows down, I hear, "We love you Kimberly!" "We love you Dave!"

We wave and wave and wave until the scene is called. I think of my best childhood friend Jenny.

Windshield wipers are rendered useless as we drive away in a sweet, teary blur.

CHAPTER 28

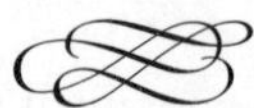

On our first leg home, Dave and I ride a car ferry across Lake Michigan. Once again, dizziness disappears—passive motion still my current best friend—and I'm swallowed into the deepest sleep in months. I recline and surrender. As eyes drift close, the last four days patch themselves into four decades, shape-shifting nature into an updated nurture; REM back-stitches wide loops between past and present, mending holes, reinforcing frayed seams.

Memories stand still: Looking out over Crystal Lake, sand under toes motionless. Sitting on Lake Winnebago's shallow floor, body rooted. Huddling over photos of family I've never known, album pages steady. Posing for camera with family I've always known, embraces sturdy.

The present is also still: A body exhilarated and exhausted, undone, finally at rest. As the Lake Michigan ferry cuts through silver waters, delicate vestibular nerves reach out and perceive true, aquatic motion. The command center, too, can rest—reorganizing, recharging, resetting. Four days and four decades of "cobwebs" clearing, new threads now spinning and stitching.

~~***Improve. Heal. Self-actualize.***~~ I am enough.

~~***Focus on the positive.***~~ All feelings are welcome.

~~***If you believe it you can achieve it.***~~ I'm not in control.

~~***Everything happens for a reason.***~~ Life doesn't need to make sense.

Four hallowed hours later, the boat approaches Wisconsin and a familiar coping strategy returns, quieter but not entirely erased by glymphatic flushing:

When the boat docks, the dizziness will be gone. All my symptoms were simply an identity reorganizing. Now, I have completed the journey, I am healed. Joseph Campbell would be proud—I accepted the quest, sailed into the tempest, slayed cthulhu monsters, and now return victoriously to solid ground.

but when the ferry docks
waves crash ashore
and follow me home

MAY 21, 2015

Dear Charlie,

I'm writing this from the ferry, somewhere between Michigan and Wisconsin, hoping the water will settle what solid ground never can. Maybe if I surrender to the rhythm, my body will remember how to be still. Maybe I will.

I think of your ride—the one you wrote about. A train rattling through the night, smoke rising, your mind dissolving into the clatter of the rails. You said that helplessness passed easily: / into sweet / effortless / peace / like they say about drowning

I can't stop thinking about that line.

You didn't know what was coming. But I do. The water. The cold. The slipping under. You wrote of drowning as if it were a surrender, as if peace could be found in the letting go. Did you still believe that when the waves took you?

And here I am, on my own ride. A cross-water vessel instead of a rackety boxcar. My body sways, my mind loops threads from an aquatic now through memories of a steadier past. But the ferry moves forward regardless, carrying me where it will.

And I understand, now, what you meant.

Nothing can be done to stop this all.

So like your blue-smoke ride—and the foreshadowed blue-watered one—I am helpless. Then allowing. Then at peace.

Like they say about healing.

CHAPTER 29

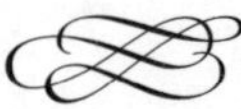

Reality strikes damning red ink through Joseph Campbell's Hero's Journey, mocking linear, rational, redemption arcs. I've failed.

Career, friendship, agency, sanity, confidence—everything falls away. I can no longer look at screens, any screen, even my phone sends nerves barreling. Watching films—once Dave's and my favorite end-of-day unwind—now sensory overload; my brain dispatches buckets of adrenaline to fight perceived danger.

I isolate, hide, and rarely leave the house. And when I do, I am a toddler clutching Dave's hand, unsure of gravity and my fraught relationship to it. More adrenaline spills out as the sidewalk interrogates my assumptions—upright, solid and reliable, now akimbo, liquid, and unsound.

Late summer, I finally meet with a neurologist—Portland's leading "dizzy doc." I enter his office certain he has an answer. Hope is hard—I've been carrying it in my pocket for months, the possibility of this doctor not having answers is inconceivable, crushing. After listening to me convey, for what feels like the hundredth time, all my bizarre experiences and sensations, he orders two days of extensive testing at Legacy Hospital's Vestibular Lab.

"It's not going to be fun, I'll tell you this right now. But we may get some answers."

I nod, obligingly. I'm quick to tell a doctor he's right or she's helping me even when I feel like I'm dying inside. I project all my absent father issues on male physicians. *Maybe he'll think I'm so smart and so sweet that he'll go the extra mile to make sure I get better. He'll look forward to the day when he sees me out in the world succeeding and think, "I helped her." He'll be proud of me.*

He was right. Two days of vestibular tests—designed to put maximum stress on all the visual and auditory connections to one's inner balance—are not fun. He was also right to use the conditional verb "may," leaving room for no answers at all.

"Kim, you passed your tests with flying colors. Your vestibular system is working great!"

Ordinarily this kind of daddy high-five would projectile-shoot glitter from my eyes. But instead, I'm deflated and in disbelief.

"So that's it? But what do I have? Are you saying nothing is wrong with me?" *Maybe I haven't conveyed how dire this is. Maybe I try too hard to look okay, to be pleasing. I can't go on like this. Does he think I'm making it all up?*

"You may have cervicogenic vertigo."

Cervic what? It takes me a moment to realize he's not talking about my vagina.

"I'll prescribe you twelve sessions with a great vestibular PT—she'll work on your neck—and you may feel some improvement. And if that doesn't work, we can start drug-trials. Benzos, anti-seizure drugs, anti-anxiety drugs. They have side-effects that you're not going to like though."

Contempt smolders inside me. *I may feel some improvement? You don't even have a definitive diagnosis?* I can barely hear him anymore as he rattles off drug names, possible complications, dependencies. He starts to read my face. I'm no longer speaking, only shuddering.

With an attempt to comfort me, he says "A tincture of time."

I stand up; the floor trampolines. He reaches out his hand and my misinterpreting heart leaps toward it—a gesture of warmth and support delivered on a scribbled RX for Diazepam.

"The body heals itself and doctors take the credit," he chuckles as I walk out the door.

I hate his flippant remark and the kernel of truth it suggests. Time can be the ultimate healer, at least in the more broad sense of healing—the kind of healing or "post-traumatic growth" that may not cure bodies but can sometimes heal spirits—a person becoming more virtuous, more *brave*, more connected because of illness or tragedy.

But I don't want my spirit to grow. I want to be fixed.

I wobble home thinking about his parting words. *If this is true, are all treatments, protocols and dollars spent along the way, just buying time? Time is also the ultimate killer. What if time makes things worse? Not everyone has access to resources and support; sometimes time destroys us.*

I recall a story Dave once shared about fishing. In his youth, he and his grandpa would bait and drop lines at the same time, but Dave never caught the first fish. One day he asked "Why do you always get first catch?" To which his grandpa replied, "Because you're not holding your mouth right." So Dave studied the old man's mouth, somedays more clenched, somedays slack, mimicking the countenance. Sometimes it worked, sometimes it didn't. But if it did, Dave attributed it to the shape he held his mouth.

Is this all healing is? A misattribution of causality? I examine each day under a microscope. If I wake up one morning and feel slightly less dizzy? It was the broccoli. And the next, if I feel worse? The pillow. More sensitive to light? The weather, Pluto squaring Disney, solar flares. I scrutinize each scenario, identifying the reason for my malaise and grasp at answers to my salvation.

I search, seek, chase—the illusion of a fix never further than the shape I hold my mouth. But the pursuit compounds the suffering. I am stuck inside a Chinese finger trap of my own making. After six weeks of strain-counter-strained hope, the physical therapist—questioning whether cervicogenic vertigo is even the culprit—sends me on my dizzy way, no better than the day I started.

Surrender and defeat vie with each other in stifling shades of grey.

I resort to spending my days in the cushioned kitchen nook—dim lighting, upholstered foam, dampened sound—a safe place for my now unbecoming life to retreat and unbecome. I insulate myself against the life I once knew and wait. First, swaddling myself with darkness, and eventually, wool.

An old Christmas gift stashed away, the *Beginner's Guide to Needle Felting* invites me into a lasting distraction from symptoms. A fiber art of the most rudimentary form, I repetitively pierce wool fibers with a sharp, barbed needle, matting loose fibers into solid shapes. Maybe it's the repetition of needlework, or wool's warm, muffled mass in hand, but I lose myself in it—for days, weeks, months, and eventually years. The cushion under me doesn't stop moving, walls continue their undulations, but the process helps drown it out so I don't, I can't, stop. Needle felting throws me a lifeline just as I'm about to go under. I hold on, each shape giving purpose and flesh to the thin-skinned vulnerability I can't express and no one can see.

With a scary phase of heavy-hitting drug trials in my treatment future, I instead head to Colorado to follow an alternative lead. I pack a few changes of clothes, some wool, a replenished bucket of hope. I plan to bunk at Mom's for ten days.

CHAPTER 30

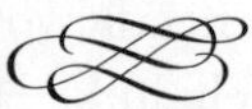

I STAY SEVEN MONTHS. I am forty years old and living with my mom. Take that, pride. Take that, overachieving perfectionist.

But I don't care. The din of dizziness doesn't leave room for me to care. I am in survival mode and in Mom's hearth, I wait out the storm.

When desperation grows, she listens without judgement. When failed treatments crush hope, she keeps believing. With my head in her lap, her hands cradling the commotion, she summons healing. Our relationship waxes bright as my identity and relevance wane into nothingness.

I am an ouroboros, eating my existence within the renewing embrace of the feminine.

But am I healing or hiding? Dave and Syd are back home, but home is now haunted—our individual and shared pain re-traumatizing each other. Lost at sea, I need Mom's particular brand of confidence, grace and unwavering optimism. I need her to make decisions for me. I need her to dream for me. With identity now blasted open, I do what is safe and familiar—I look to Mom to build my narrative.

Mom's intelligence, love and marked magnetism are a dwelling for many. For as long as I can remember, she's presented with polished, but sincere, optimism; uncertainty and negativity digested in her sleep by a dependable shadow gobbler. By morning, the chaos is sorted, the meaning clear. In my youth, while tentative frames of my own forming identity would montage into meaninglessness, it felt a lot more safe to buy her narrative than to discover and write my own.

Her truth was a snow globe that never stopped snowing—divine beauty and perfection blurred the plastic, paint-chipped faces of children on skates. I didn't want my life to settle into a meaningless made-in-China export. Standing inside the globe, Mom's narrative swirled around my head, obscuring my own truth, and it was glorious.

But now the snow is settling, and I'm unmoored by the broken bits, the hard faces, the scenes ordinary and void of meaning.

Occasionally Mom encourages an outing, to say small yeses in my new life defined by *no.* Most evenings I retreat to bed after dinner or sit at the dining room table poking needles into wool until eyes grow heavy. On a rare night, I'll "watch" a movie—mask over eyes and volume so low I can barely decipher dialog. But I'm feeling brave tonight so I venture out—*an experiment!*—with Mom to see the indie film *Unbranded,* a documentary that follows four men and sixteen mustangs on an epic 3,000-mile journey from Mexico to Canada.

Mom is running her usual fifteen minutes late so only a few front row seats remain open in the theater. We walk through the dark, the equine stampede deafening. I breathe into my diaphragm, *I am safe, I am safe,* but already know it's too much. My sweaty hands clench the armrests, a knee-jerk attempt to stabilize haphazard signaling. The screen looms, a suspended tsunami just seconds from impact, towering over my cowering existence. And even though the edits are mercifully well-paced, the blow-out-your-eardrums Cinemax experience is enough assault for all my senses combined.

I am desperate to have a successful outing, to feel normal again, to not ruin the evening. So I endure all one hour and forty-six minutes of the terrordome. I am a pool of sweat when the credits roll. The floor drops out under each step as we make our way back to the car. Mom notes my distress, but not its magnitude.

When we return to the safety of her townhouse, I immediately drop to the floor, pressing myself into solid, hardwood feedback, something to settle the eight-hundred pinballs all firing at once in my brain. The floor jolts up and down, side to side, a zigzag herky-jerky patternless motion all the more pronounced by indisputable stillness. I so badly want out of my experience. I must, but can't, escape my body. Our experiment was a failure; I'm a failure. While Mom reviews the movie, "Incredible scenery…" "The masculine test of endurance…" "In wildness is the preservation of…" somewhere from the periphery of embodiment, fury collapses in, and then explodes out of me. I stand up, two feet from her face and scream,

"SHUUUUUUUUTTTTTTTTT UPPPPPPPPPPPP!!!!!!!!"

Both stunned, we stand in silence.

And then, an unfamiliar sight—a jaw trembles, tears well, snow settles. But instead of reaching out to her, I march out of the room. I am full of indignation I can't comprehend. Rage eviscerates rationality.

I collapse on the guest room bed, staring at a ceiling I've memorized. *How dare I? Mom, patient as ever, takes my blows without protest, yet because of my stupid reaction to a stupid movie, I lashed out at her. I'm the one I should be angry at—for not leaving the theater, for pushing myself too far. It's not her job to protect me. So why does it feel like it is?*

Her beautiful face, drained of color, her tears, her unsteady jaw—I clench my own as the images loop through me. I don't want to stay angry; I crave peace, even more so with its biological absence. I hurt her and I need to make it right.

I get up. Walk back to the kitchen.

Her back is to me, perched on a red stool, casually munching leftovers while MSNBC hums in the background. As if nothing happened. Mom has a dial embedded in her brain, I'm sure of it—some innate mechanism that allows her to flip in and out of emotional states with ease. I envy this in her. She welcomes the biting edge of relationship, the moments of truth that shatter boundaries and invite intimacy. She has an almost super-human, infinite trust in the unfolding of events. She knows we will find each other again.

I take a breath, step forward.

"I'm sorry."

It doesn't need to be spelled out—I'm pissed about my situation. Unscrewing the valve and letting off steam sometimes is necessary; but rage is scary and threatens abandonment.

Months pass and the outbursts arrive more frequently. She doesn't abandon.

I never plan for them to happen, erupting without warning. My adult self can't rationalize away the child's fury. *YOU WERE SUPPOSED TO PROTECT ME*, she screams—not back in the movie theater, but forty years ago when I first shaped the word *DAD*. I ask her to tell "the Charlie story" over and over again, trying to understand her choice to stay in the dark.

I explode again. We hug. I explode again. We cry. I explode again. We talk through it. This thawing business is a slushy mess. Mom's shadow gobbler is fat and her brain's emotional dial is getting a workout.

And then, I hear it. Soft, but differentiating consonants free our tangled branches; tiny shoots push down, down, down from my feet.

Her beautiful, glassy eyes are inches from mine—vulnerable but certain, "I'm so sorry Kim, I'm so sorry I didn't protect you, that I didn't pursue the truth. I was so focused on keeping everything together, I was afraid to find out the truth and risk everything falling apart."

I hear "sorry," I hear "pursue truth," but it's the everyday "you" —incarnate and valid—that fortifies and repairs. The snow globe shatters; I no longer identify as an accessory to her story. I am not the neat epilogue to her choices. I am an individual—with my own needs, my own desires, my own failures. Someone who was protected *from* the truth, not protected *by* the truth. Someone who didn't get to decide her own story because it was edited and tidied up before she was even born. And now I get to.

We hold each other. I feel no blame, only deep, undying love for the woman *now* and also the woman *then* who did her very best to protect me from hurt, only to discover forty years later that the truth can hurt, but it also can heal. It *does* hurt. It *does* heal.

* * *

With each passing month, I feel less and less Joseph Campbell's hero and more a failed mortal drowning in the River Styx, trapped soulless between life and afterlife. But cathartic shifts with Mom are a healing balm so magical thinking interjects with dire conviction: *Mom's apology was the missing piece. Now the journey is complete and the dizziness will surely go away.*

But time has other plans.

Cycles of optimism and disappointment mock my unflagging pursuit of a cure. Mom tirelessly keeps believing. Dave and I limp along with the distance and his helplessness furthers the strain. We nearly break-up multiple times, giving up on each other, giving up on ourselves. In Boulder, Colorado—the capital of toxic positivity—I am drowning in a sea of sanguinity. Everyone has an answer, a cure or knows someone who was cured. *But why not me?* I am the unchosen one. The harder I chase, the worse it gets. I crave stillness so badly—now seven months, 24/7, of maddening motion—my body has *vanished, disappeared, gone missing.*

I want to give up.

I start praying. Hard. With no real religious compass, I'm not sure to whom, but I fall to my knees anyway and go on a deity shopping spree.

A psychic says my "spiritual body has a miasma" and it will take five months to dissipate. I count the days dutifully. I go to her psychic cleansing sessions. I repeat her mantras. An acupuncturist gives me a copper Quan Yin plate to put under my pillow. I pray to her before bed and then curse her in the middle of night after sleepless night. I practice Qi Gong. I meditate. I read Mooji, Adyashanti, Krishnamurti, anyone who ends their name in "i." I reread Pema Chodrin's *When Things Fall Apart.* I create a Mother Mary shrine on my bed stand.

The following February I return home to Portland to attend a defense attorney's scheduled mediation, the entrails of the 2014 bike incident still dragging behind me. Insurance wanted to settle right after the accident but I was advised to wait until all medical treatment had been completed. Now, two years post-accident, I'm still in the thick of it. The optometrist says it's my eyes. The ENT says it's my ears. The physical therapist says it's my pelvis. The neurologist says it's my neck. The psychiatrist says it's trauma. The psychic says it's my dirty soul.

So the settlement drags on. Returning to an eight-hour deposition is no warm homecoming. But in hindsight, though as dizzy as the day I left, I'm glad law intervenes and flies what's left of me back to Dave.

I ache for the loss of our life. One wobbly step at a time, I try to stay focused on moments of gratitude—our stubborn love despite the heartache, the birds singing at sunrise, the sweet potato on my plate. If I zoom out, I fall into a hole of self-pity. *I am forty-one going on eighty.* The invisibility of symptoms and lack of diagnosis compound the ache. Friends and coworkers eventually stop asking questions and I stop talking about it. There's nothing to say except *I don't know. I don't know, I don't know. I don't know.*

But at the end of each day, someone lies by my side. And even though my sleep is more fitful than his, my psyche leans in and listens. She's strangely comforted, even relieved, by his way. Dave isn't trying to fix me. He's just being with me.

His energy is heavy, sure, and undoubtedly tangled in unprocessed trauma, but fathering a daughter with intellectual disability for twenty-one years has taught him to be in relationship to *what is*, and not *what might be*. Being next to him, I inch slowly—ever so slowly—closer to myself *as I am.*

One afternoon Dave returns home with an old, thrift store painting of a ship at sea. The sails are full and taut as the dark tempest threatens to swallow the ship whole. As I study the acrylic likeness of my experience, my beloved atheist—still drawing from decades of Fundamentalist Baptist conditioning—offers a parable about Christ at sea during a large squall. While his disciples are physically sick from the swells and gripped with fear for their lives, Christ lies on the bow of the ship and sleeps.

HE LIES ON THE BOW OF THE SHIP AND SLEEPS.

This image becomes my anchor. Daily, hourly, I close my eyes, paint myself onto the bow, imagine feeling so safe, so trusting, that I can finally let go and rest. I stop wishing for a cure and start envisioning peace in the storm. And most days, I'm baffled—surrendering completely to my symptoms and allowing them to run their course feels implausible. It's like trying to undo millions of years of biological hardwiring: when a threat is perceived, fight it, fix it, flee from it. I find little relief, but unlike everything else I've tried, this practice puts me in relationship to myself, exactly as I am, not some distant *possible* me once I'm cured. The phrase itself—*once I'm cured*—now suddenly feels presumptuous.

I am told Grandmother Isabelle, Charlie's mom, died reading one of her favorite passages, Psalm 38:21–22. One minute she was upright at the breakfast table with the Bible open in her hands, the next, she was gone. The passage closes with a prayer: *Lord, give us the peace that passeth all understanding, and the understanding that gives us peace.*

I want to learn, I need to learn, to live with an unconditional peace despite the circumstances of my body, my life. If repose and happiness are tethered to an endless continuum of pain, relief, disappointment, and hope, I'm signing up for misery. And though it feels irrational if not impossible to feel tranquil during a shit storm, and never experiencing stillness again unfathomable, I carry Dave's painting and Grandma Isabelle's passage within me until the incomprehensible becomes imaginable, and the possibility that frightens me most becomes my very doorway into peace.

CHAPTER 31

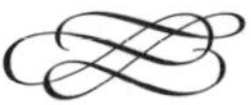

UNDER THE CARE of a new physician—one of Oregon's most respected naturopaths who "likes complicated cases"—I begin to feel buoyed, not pummeled, for the first time in two years. True to the naturopathic approach, Dr. Vickers doesn't target the dizziness directly—she, like my growing list of practitioners, has no diagnosis — but instead, slowly, judiciously, supports my whole system—balancing thyroid hormones, regulating sleep, identifying inflammation factors, and releasing the fascial grip in my head and neck from two years of bracing against constant movement.

It's not immediate, and I arrive at her clinic in tears more times than I care to admit, but slowly, timidly, I feel a shift. Pairing her intuitive and skillful approach with my newfound practice to find "peace that passeth understanding," I begin to grow a spaciousness around the dizziness and my gripping resistance to it. The unsteadiness doesn't go away, or even diminish most days, but just as a clear, blue sky is always above the grayest clouds, a pervasive sense of calm starts to hold the constant oscillation. Two unlikely companions—stillness and movement—learn compatibility.

I challenge myself to take more risks—small, calculated risks—and say yes more than no. Like the still-fragile shoots of spring, each yes a reaching memory of sun, and the sunniness of reaching. Each experience a welcoming, not a regret. I meet a friend for an hour. Dave and I eat out at a favorite taqueria. I venture to Powell's Books. And even though I often pay for it, my nervous system over-stimulated from habitual under-stimulus, the little wins build courage within the monotony of eat-needle wool-walk-sleep. I've become a REALLY. BORING. PERSON but allowing, instead of fighting, my pared-down existence creates the safety my brain needs to finally rest and adapt. I don't know if I'm healing, but I am learning to live inside the not-knowing.

* * *

Syd starts attending a day program at a large, private home in Washington for adults with disabilities. Offering intellectually diverse individuals an independent, community-based experience, the facility intimates a brighter future for Syd. Our hearts are tentative though; having hope is a lot harder than having none.

Dave and I practice patience—with ourselves and each other—there is so much to process, too much, and neither have the foundational strength yet to face the collision of emotions head-on. We do what we can in the meantime. We wait, we watch, we stretch, and we submit as best we can while taking small steps forward. The future is still unformed, still unsettled, but for now, we lean into what's in front of us. Our enduring love allows for time to rebuild, and that alone, rebuilds.

I also need to sell my house. My income hovers near zero and happy, domestic memories of years past are buried under the dank flotsam of two years at sea. Our bedroom is littered with abandoned prayers. Mirrors discard a face no longer recognizable. Dave and I need more than a fresh coat of paint over our heartache; we need a new shared hearth.

So when we receive a wedding invite from Cousin Greta, enough little yeses inspire a bigger RSVP-YES. It will be a great opportunity to meet more of the Brauer clan and to reconnect with those already in my heart. Our communications are regular now. Not a week or two passes without some sort of hello: a snap of a recent snowstorm or spring flowers with a string of heart emojis, a letter or package in the mail, a phone call, and Rich's favorite (and my least), FaceTime. But I cave, always surprised by how easy it feels...with him.

Without deliberate planning, we have become family.

SEPTEMBER 2, 2015

Dear Charlie,

I've been thinking about homes and the rooms they contain.

The ones we enter, the ones we leave behind. The ones that keep us waiting. You wrote about June passing into a two-room dimension—one where all things lost reside—fountain pens, marbles, sweaters—and another, vast as the sky, filled with friendships, experiences, and firsts. Some things vanish for good, misplaced in the small room. Others remain, waiting in the expanse of the second, untouched by time, held for us until we are ready to return.

I wonder if that's what's happening to me now. If I've spent years searching in the wrong room. Grasping at the small things—control, certainty, answers—while the truths that have shaped me, the ones I feared, the ones I thought I had to leave behind, have been waiting all along.

What if loss isn't an ending, but a keeping place? What if the things we resist—grief, uncertainty, brokenness, vulnerability—don't disappear but simply wait, gathering quiet strength? They live in the body like breath. The inhale, tight and unrelenting. The exhale, the opening, the becoming.

I've spent so much of my life in the inhale. Bracing. Fighting. Clutching at what I could name, what I want, what I could fix. But I think I'm beginning to understand what you meant. That the deepest, most ineffable things—what we love, what we've rejected, what we've lost—lie patiently in waiting.

And when we finally exhale, they don't just return. They complete us.

Maybe that's what grace is.

Not an answer, not an escape. Just the moment we allow ourselves to become whole.

CHAPTER 32

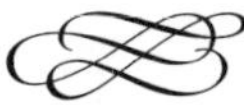

Dave and I plan our return to the Midwest for Greta's wedding, but instead of flying conveniently into Chicago, we route tickets to Milwaukee—there's a place I need to visit in Ferryville, Wisconsin.

A year ago, on a whim, I wrote a letter to the owners of Charlie's hand-built, two-story cottage. To my surprise, they replied with uncommon enthusiasm to connect.

Purchased in the early 2000s from a previous owner, Dan and Diana Chandler lovingly restored Charlie's home, turning it into a treasured family retreat. When we first spoke on the phone, I was overcome by their kindness—generously offering time, stories and an invitation to visit the house and surrounding seventy-nine acres whenever convenient. Charlie's original investment was a much smaller plot, but his love for history and charming affinity for older generations turned his thirty-plus acres into almost eighty when elderly neighbors up and down the valley deeded land to him upon their deaths.

The Chandlers also described Charlie's flawless woodwork and his unusual penchant for marking his existence in hidden corners—on cupboards, door frames and secret nooks. Charlie left engraved epitaphs everywhere.

And not just in his home. There was the chest of drawers he

carved into before leaving for basic training during the Vietnam War: ***1969 Michigan—San Diego navy base. I never wanted to go.***

...and inside his homemade guitar: ***In commemoration of campout #12 in the hills of Tennessee by Chuck and Dave, August 8, 1970***

...and scrawled on the back of Paul McCartney's album *Ram*: ***Just words, like all of us.***

Did Charlie ever intend for his messages to surface?

Am I one of his epitaphs written in flesh?

When I text Diana about our plans to return to the Midwest for a wedding, she replies with enthusiasm, assuring me that the property is looking more beautiful than ever, still glowing from their daughter's wedding reception there over the summer. But a week before our flight, a major storm hits. Torrential rains fall for nine days. The Mississippi floods. Mudslides close the main highway. Houses slip off bluffs and onto the road. And more rain is coming.

Fearing the worst, Diana sends me an update. Rush Creek, which runs through their property and feeds into the Mississippi, is rising fast. I suggest we cancel our visit, but she refuses. The storm threatens to wash away her own world, but she refuses to let it take mine.

She apologizes in advance for the damage, for not being able to show me Charlie's home exactly as she'd envisioned. She writes, "I wanted everything to be perfect for you, so you could see how special your dad was, why he loved this place so much. But you will still see it—just look beyond the mess. Your daddy would be so proud of you. I know I am."

Sometimes the kindness of strangers feels less like social propriety and more celestial intervention. I am the protagonist in a magical realism mystery novel. *Am I the author or is someone else writing me into these scenes?*

When we arrive at our VRBO in Wisconsin, I spread-eagle beneath Dave and try as I might to alight into gravity. One long flight plus an equally long drive deliver a troop of hyperactive chimps into my brain. But things are different, now.

Now, I am armed. I have my second-by-second practice of

surrendering to what is. Unlike many other abandoned meditation hacks, I now have a visceral opportunity to master letting go, in perpetuity.

Twenty-four hours later, the dizziness settles down, only a few rowdy chimps remaining.

And twenty-four hours after that, I learn my house sells. DocuSign makes it easy; letting go of the house, even easier. I listen to torrential rain on the roof, washing away homes and their memories within, and wonder what else needs to be released.

On Sunday morning we awaken to a cloudless, blue sky. The Mississippi's now lazy, swollen current belies its cruel potential. Diana calls with a plan, "Let's meet at The Wooden Nickel, a hole-in-the-wall in Ferryville, and then you can follow us in on the washed-out gravel road. It's too dangerous to go it alone." *Do I detect tears in her voice?* We offer our help—shoveling mud, sponging down walls, making trips to the dump, meals, anything to soften the blow. My own excitement to visit Charlie's home is a discomfiting contrast to their monumental tragedy. I remind myself: *This isn't Charlie's home anymore. This is the Chandlers' home.*

When we finally exchange hugs in the bar's parking lot, tears threaten another flood, and we follow them in on Rush Creek Road.

The damage is astonishing. The creek has torn itself a wide and violent path right up to the house, eroding and pitting decades of family memories; thick layers of squelchy mud and sediment now carpet a once-idyllic scape; jagged green islands of lawn overstate impermanence. Trees are horizontal. A propane tank rests two hundred yards away in a field of muddy corn. A six-foot deep, gaping hole—where flooding water formed a hydraulic and exploded the sump pump—carves into the basement, now four-feet deep with earth. I take it all in under a gentle autumn sun while wrens trill indifference.

After a thorough tour—our grief-struck tour guides still taking time to showcase Charlie's craftsmanship—the four of us take a break outside and assess next steps. The water damage in the house is irreparable. The property, ravaged. The basement needs to be filled and sealed. While the Chandlers weigh their grim options, Dave and I stand near—perplexing bystanders to another's immediate tragedy. The ground wavers beneath me. Rush Creek has stopped flooding but its specter still rocks my bones.

Then Diana looks at me, eyes brimming,

"Kimberly, what if we have to raze the property?"

The direction of her question puzzles me, like she's asking Charlie's permission, through me. *Once erased by a massive force of water, is Charlie now tidying up loose ends? Maybe he doesn't want crumbs of his existence around anymore.*

When Diana's question lands into the solemn circle of our bodies, every hair on my arms stands on end in epiphany—this isn't a meeting, this is a memorial.

And Charlie, carried in on the same elemental power that took him away, offers his final epitaph. Not with knife or hardwood surface, just water. And lots of it.

Let go.

* * *

A week before Dave and I move out, let go, of our home, an invisible rotor rooter snakes its way through our lives. Within the same twenty-four hours, Dave's mom dies, we put our beloved twenty-one year-old Kitty Pang down, and a few blocks away, an entire building blows up. When the gas-leak explosion happens, I am full of acupuncture needles, lying in repose, and then not. My ears ring and the clinic windows answer while staff run around in the dark— though clueless of the cause—reassuring patients. I lie unsure if the blast is real or just the force of my own life—two-and-a-half years of upheaval, disorientation, catharsis and adaptation—combusting under the pressure of one incarnation.

My home now echoes without furniture, shedding its namesake after ninety-percent of our belongings are sold or donated. King Fred, the scruffy, feral stray we've been feeding and loving for four years stands at the back door—he is the hardest to leave behind. As I scrub cupboards and counters, I open the back door, inviting him in to unfamiliar territory. His recurring mange didn't inspire an open door policy; but now, who cares? He's tentative but laps around the kitchen island a few times and then bolts to his outdoor kingdom. Before we depart, we kneel at the back door and give him a last goodbye, a chin scratch, a stroke on the head. He cocks his snaggle-tooth mouth upwards and coos with his awkward, "I love this but fuck off." The house holds stories and memories but this black, block-headed beast holds the key. He was the predictable groundskeeper, reminding us in the last two-and-a-half years of strife, that a little food, shelter and kindness can be enough. He is the sage embodiment of living unfixed, every sunbaked or rain-soaked inch of fur a reminder of Lao Tzu's teaching: *Be content with what you have; rejoice in the way things are. When you realize there is nothing lacking, the whole world belongs to you.* We give his cat house to a neighbor along with monthly cash for food so his boundless life chasing chipmunks remains unbound.

After closing the front door for the last time, we sit in our packed car, motionless. We know little about what's next; with everything we need behind us—two small suitcases, a few bins with essential documents, a computer, and a duffle bag of colorful wool—we are headed to the Oregon coast to rent our friend's property for seven months and buy time until "what's next" is clear. When Dave turns the ignition, our eyes brim with tears, less a sadness of goodbye and more a wet, cellular emptying. Tears exhume any last attachment and wash it into the void, hollowing a shelter for something new.

We drive west along the Sunset Highway, our emptiness opening her mouth to wilderness. Like the winding rural lines before us, our life's narrative now meanders and bends with unpredictability.

Dave and I build on today, tomorrow still an uncertainty. Our home of over a decade is no more. I haven't worked in two-and-a-half years. My family has grown beyond comprehension. And my sense of self—unformed—is now taking shape as pieces of my biological foundation fall into place. Holding them in my hands, I step back and see not just the puzzle they complete, but the hollow space they once occupied. They take up space now, and with their certainty, so do I.

But the paradox of a self more-defined is that she is then free to undefine. As I incarnate, magical thinking gives way to magical presence—a state of solidarity and wonder not for what could be, but with what is. And like the water under my feet, *what is* changes, moment, by moment, by moment—the details of an identity drops of rain in a bestowing, ancient origin.

When Dave and I pull into the sleepy, coastal town of Manzanita, a cloth of orange over the Pacific shrouds our past in dying light. We stop the car, roll down the windows and breathe it in. The ground shifts back and forth under me. Dave doesn't feel it but I do. I'm becoming used to this sensation; I'm becoming better at allowing; I'm becoming unconcerned with becoming. I'm also getting used to my two dads. One I never knew, one I adored, both a longing. The ground will solidify someday. Or maybe it won't. But its constant, liquid teaching is a foundation from which I will unbuild the rest of my life.

With Dave's hand in mine, we watch the sun relax into the horizon. Tomorrow its arc of almost will rise over the hills, the animals scurrying into light, the sunflowers turning to watch. Feeling the sun's arrival rise above my own body of water, I celebrate this wild, untamable life.

MARCH 30TH, 2019

Dear Charlie,

Dave and I live on a farm in rural Oregon. Today, I spent the afternoon barefoot, toes pressing down firmly into the Willamette Valley's rich, loamy soil. Our driveway is winding, the curves unhurried, the sky hooded with cherry blossoms and maple leaf buds, and the wind delivers a promising return beyond the green tunnel; the crunch of gravel, reminding me of your own home-stretch sounds of promise and return, bending my perception of time and place.

/ this small habit born of a simple need / which, natural and unprompted, ties them together / across the bounds of death, and across time /

The early spring sun is cool but knows herself and where she's headed. I know that I am here, not where I'm headed. The ground beneath me dips and sways; my body grips, then allows. Five years of discovery still integrating, discomfort becoming my new comfortable.

You once wondered / is it possible / to leave a part of me behind / (you ask / which part?) / but what takes its place / and these parts / strewn over time and space / in houses / hearts / on hillsides / stages / or paper / are more than / hubcaps along a freeway?

And to that I reply: Your devoted intimacy with life is more than a hubcap. Inscribed on page or strummed through fingers or witnessed with gentle attention, your written, spoken and sung truth didn't roll into a ditch but instead landed in me; a lasting song that reminded and awakened my own.

Now, we sing it together.

CHAPTER 33

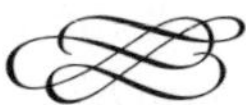

IT'S MIDNIGHT. Five years ago I opened an email from 23andMe and my sense of self changed forever. Tonight, I stand at a bathroom mirror, splashing off the heat of a July sun. Dave and I are in Michigan with the Brauer family. It's a family tradition to gather at the cottage around the fourth of July and now, two years and counting, it is ours. The cool water feels good on my sunburned skin. I close my eyes and listen to it sing past my ears, a soundtrack to the montage of faces and new memories crowding my brain—

Lanky nieces and nephews hurling themselves off the dock with the same abandon I know in my own limbs.

My great aunt Lois (who insists I call her "grandma") and her gentle, teary embrace, "What a blessing to experience you at the end of my life."

Dave's question to Rich, "What was your first thought after you read Kimberly's initial outreach?"

And Rich's reaching hand across a pitcher of margaritas to grab mine in response,

"I wanted it to be true."

I turn off the faucet, dry my face with a towel and then it hits me. Staring into the mirror, feet solidly planted on the bath mat, everything changes. A lightning bolt insight—but instead of descending from an abstract sky, the thought comes from my flesh. The ground under my feet shifts—liquid to solid. Moments later it will return to liquid, to the same unexplained, undiagnosed dizziness that still eludes every doctor. But in this singular, steady, anchored moment, words—shaped from ancient synapses descending from the pads of my feet—form themselves into a thought. *I am a Brauer.*

I've had this thought before, I tell myself. *So why is it different this time? Has it taken my cells five years to finally get it?* Like a sticky name tag, edges bent up and caught in my hair, my new identity has been less than skin deep. It was a thought, a fact, cut from a DNA test result and pasted into my brain. My cells didn't know what to do with it; they needed time and the slow metabolism of seasons to comprehend and assimilate.

Quietly, the thought presses into my flesh. I stare at my wet reflection in the mirror and call out to Dave to tell him the news.

"Dave, I'm a Brauer."

It's not a headline anymore. It's just a sentence—one of many—that I've clutched tightly in my fist for a lifetime. I've been gripping this story like a script, desperate to find in its lines the definitive version of me. A Brauer. A Warner. A daughter. A seeker. A mystery. Each label a sentence, each sentence a grasp at coherence.

But eventually, my hold grows tired and sweaty. The paper softens, the ink bleeds.

So I loosen my grip.

open to the sun
ink fades
exposed to the rain
words smudge
stanzas underlined—
underrated
words crossed out—
cross over

. . .

unfolding
i understand
unfixed
i am
not the dancer
but the stage
less the word
more the page

EPILOGUE

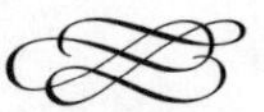

Now, I approach my body, myself, with curiosity. I stand on the precipice of a new way of being, and I question:

Can we experience purposeful, meaningful lives when we're in pain? Can wellness include illness, disability and limitation? Do we need to always be improving, actualizing, reaching, and seeking, to be fully living? Is it possible that our grief, fallibility, failure, limitation, impermanence and brokenness are actually the very experiences that save us?

What are the waves like today? Am I on a river or an ocean? What parts of my body are tensing around the sensation? What parts are chill and going along for the ride?

I notice and allow the waves to crash under and around me. Sometimes they even increase in intensity for a spell as I pour my full awareness into them. But I stay curious, open. The sensations don't change, but my relationship to them changes.

The waves aren't bad or good, they simply exist. But they are not all that exists.

And then ever so slowly, without expectation or urgency, something new eventually arrives—a twin of sorts—an abiding, calm, awareness that surrounds and imbues the experience with quiet stillness. Not a stillness that erases the sensations, but one that holds them. A "spiritual stillness" if you will—effortless, peaceful and most notably, unconditional.

Five long years after the first symptoms of dizziness began, the COVID pandemic swept across the planet and telemedicine became a standard for care. This enabled me to finally consult with Dr. Shin Beh, one of the country's leading neurologists for central dizziness disorders, and receive a long-awaited diagnosis for the tempest that had descended into my brain. Within thirty minutes, he gave a name: *Mal de Débarquement Syndrome*(MdDS), also known as *Non-Motion Triggered Oscillatory Vertigo*—a rare neurological disorder uniquely identified by the temporary relief of its constant rocking, bobbing, or swaying sensations when in passive motion.

MdDS is not a psychiatric disorder, but because the vestibular and stress-response systems in the brain are closely linked, individuals who experience shock or trauma may be more susceptible to developing centrally related vestibular disorders, including MdDS, vestibular migraine and persistent postural-perceptual dizziness (PPPD). A recent study published in *Frontiers of Neurology* highlights the challenges to diagnosis and care, as well as promising treatment protocols:

To this day, MdDS is categorized as a rare disorder, although this classification may not accurately reflect the prevalence of the condition. This discrepancy arises from the significant number of individuals who remain undiagnosed due to the challenges of accurately identifying the syndrome. The prevalence of this condition has only been assessed in one study to date, where it was estimated to have an occurrence rate of 1.3 to 3% (similar to Menières disease) in a neuro-otological clinic. On average, MdDS patients undergo 19 consultations with healthcare professionals before receiving a correct diagnosis, where this diagnostic process can last several years.

Some researchers and clinicians have also noted a correlation between chronic dizziness and serotonin dysfunction—common in certain mental health disorders including Obsessive Compulsive Disorder (OCD). While I had exhibited OCD behaviors from an early age, I never considered this particular brain chemistry might have predisposed me to MdDS. One of the most effective treatments for OCD is called Exposure Ritual Prevention (ERP) therapy, which gradually introduces distressing stimuli, training the brain to respond to discomfort in healthier ways.

It is both surprising and revelatory that my own brain created the ultimate ERP therapy—constant, inescapable discomfort. My lifelong obsession with avoiding or fixing pain had led me, inevitably, to the one thing I had spent years trying to escape: surrendering to the unnerving experience of simply being in a body. And because the vestibular and stress-response centers in the brain are so deeply intertwined, the more we focus on symptoms, the more we amplify them. This is why stopping the chase for a cure became my very doorway into peace.

For so long, my relentless pursuit of control had only deepened my suffering.

The child who couldn't control her thoughts needed to know her noisy, compulsive brain was lovable and human. The teenager locked in the bathroom, picking at her skin, longed to embrace her imperfections. The young woman who froze instead of feeling, who preferred magical thinking over reality, who buried rage under a pleasing smile—she needed to welcome her feelings as wise and powerful allies. The adult who became overwhelmed by shock and grief needed to know she could survive the heat of living.

I think I can. I think I can.

And she could.

RESOURCES

If you or someone you know is struggling to understand the frightening experience of constant motion, you are not alone.

Organizations:

Vestibular Disorders Association

ADeV

Video/Audio:

Life Rebalanced Chronicles

The Steady Coach

ICU Podcast: Real Patients, Real Practitioners, Real Conversations

Talk Dizzy To Me

Meniere's Muse

Finding Joy in your Vestibular Migraine

Articles:

NYT article: Why Doctors Dismiss Dizziness

New Yorker article: Why Dizziness is Still a Mystery

Practitioners/Clinics:

Dr. Shin Beh

Johns Hopkins Neuro-Visual and Vestibular Disorders Center

Books:

The Dizzy Cook
Finding Balance
Victory Over Vestibular Migraine
The Mediterranean Migraine Diet
Disembark: Overcoming Mal de Debarquement Syndrome

ACKNOWLEDGMENTS

To thank everyone who made this book possible is to touch the deeply interwoven fabric of my life—the countless hands and hearts that held me as I became the woman capable of telling this story. What follows is a humble attempt to name those threads, though many remain unnamed but not unfelt.

BOOK CREATION ACKNOWLEDGMENTS

To my editor, Molly Zakoor, whose clarity, sensitivity, and wisdom elevated every chapter. And to Jen Violi, my early reader and local friend, who gave her time and heart to the earliest drafts before they ever saw the light of day. To Empress Editions: Alisa Kennedy Jones for shepherding this book into the world with fierce devotion and the electric intelligence of a thousand geniuses combined; for holding the vision with the grit of a triathlete and the heart of a poet. She is a one-woman society—publisher, strategist, advocate, visionary, and artist, all in one blazing force; Dr. Heather Bartos, for championing the feminine voice in publishing; and the PR team—Erinn McGrath and Eva Sikelianos—for believing this story needs to be in the world. A nod to David McLaughlin, who designed the gorgeous cover (though he never likes to take credit), and who happens to be my beloved husband—so his deeper thanks live further down.

PHYSICAL, CREATIVE & EMOTIONAL SUPPORT

Dr. Shin Beh, thank you for naming the unnamable and treating it with your extensive knowledge and experience. Dr. Edyth Vickers, your unparalleled skill and intuitive healing presence carried me through. For love and emotional ballast: my mother Nancy Warner, brother Eric Warner, sisters-in-and-out-laws Jeneye Abele-Warner, Kirsten Warner, and my beloved nephews and niece Aidan, Reid, and Raina Warner—thank you for being my heart and my hearth. And to my new clan: the Brauers and Bresemans —your love and openness to my story, our story, and bravery to let it change us, is a gift of a lifetime—one that transformed what family means to me. To Dr. Keith Slicho and Evan Manée for teaching my body to become resilient again. To Dani Shapiro: for seeing the universal in my personal, and for featuring my story on *Family Secrets*. To Dr. Annie Brewster, for introducing me to narrative medicine and becoming a kindred guide and friend. To Cynthia Ryan of the Vestibular Disorders Association: our collaborations shaped so much of my professional identity post-diagnosis. To Daniel DeFabio, for inviting me to empower others through Global Genes and the Disorder Channel. To Elizabeth Jameson, for your radiant mind and for our work on *MS Confidential*. To Dr. Moyez Jiwa, for your steadfast commitment to bettering the patient doctor relationship and inviting me to be part of the mission. To Michael Wolcott, the brilliant film editor and ally. To Gustavo Serafini, who is helping me grow Unfixed Media with faith and vision. To Sara Nesson, co-creator in movement and meaning. To JenEric—you know who you are and how much I adore you. To my earliest draft readers and your whole-hearted encouragement: Jen Violi, Greg Temple, Aunt Janet, Mom, Eric. And to Jess Stainbrook, for helping lift Unfixed Media off the ground.

INSPIRATION & INTELLECTUAL SOURCES

To the thinkers and writers whose words both root and wing my path: Allie Brosh, Andrea Gibson, Albert Camus, Dani Shapiro, Ingrid Rojas Contreras, Krista Tippett, Linda Hogan, Maria Popova, Marion Woodman, Ocean Vuong, Rachel Naomi Remen, Rebekah Taussig, Richard Powers, Robin Wall Kimmerer, Ruth Ozeki, Sarah Ramey, Sophie Strand, Wendell Berry. To the spiritual beacons: Adyashanti, Pema Chödrön, Roshi Joan Halifax and the Upaya Zen Center, Viktor Frankl, Alan Lightman.

FAMILY

I couldn’t dream of a more beloved motley crew to tumble with through this wild field of love. To Dave: my partner, my home. Thank you for never giving up, for meeting each moment without expectation, and for showing me that life doesn’t need to be fixed—its miracle is already here. Your quiet steadiness softened my striving, and your love met me exactly as I was. To Mom, Nancy Warner: you are my eternal sunshine, the embodiment of ever-renewing optimism and love. To my step-daughter, Sydney: you are the first human to bravely show me just how joyful “living unfixed” can be. And to the entire McLaughlin family for always leading with warmth and kindness. To my brother Eric Warner: my protector, my co-adventurer, my co-conspirator, my dearest friend. And to the sensational sisters he gifted me: Jeneye Abele Warner and Kirsten Warner. To the Brauer and Breseman families: I won't name names to honor your privacy, but your response to my arrival in your lives —"I wanted it to be true”—and the reception that followed echoes in my heart forever. Thank you for seeing him in me, and loving us both in the same embrace. To my two fathers: David Warner, who has always been and will forever be my soul-father. And Charles Brauer, whose creative spirit lives in me—may I forever honor your DNA’s song. 43 forever.

COMMUNITIES & INSTITUTIONS

To the Unfixed and Vestibular Communities: Thank you for letting your stories rise to the surface. In your willingness to be seen—not in spite of your symptoms, but through them—I learned how to stay soft and open inside my own. Your courage became my courage. To the cast of the original Unfixed docuseries: Alayna Allen, Rachelle Alford, Jeneye Abele, Brianna Cardenas, Bethany Cook, Stefanie Grant, Jacqueline Lily Doyle, Elizabeth Jameson, Brian Langhans, Brian Nice, Rene Morales, William Ross, Dylan Shanahan, Sofia

Krasteva, Mac Brand, Todd Vogt, Shayla VanTassel. To my vesties (the Vestibular Community) including: Rishi Bhosale, Sandy Brunner, Nicolle Cure, Johan Galeano, Lynn Johnson, David Morrill, Rupal Rajani, Steve Schwier, Alicia Wolf, Colin & Gabriela, Marissa Aldrete, Yannis, Benaniba, Paul Burnside, Heather Davies, Rochelle Matheson, Joy Mohr, Emma Rodgers, Etta and Mike Sundberg, Kevin Thomas. To my Substack readers—you held me, cheered me on, and reminded me that I was never writing into a void. With deep gratitude, I name you: Adam Nathan, Alisa Kennedy Jones, Allegra Huston, Allison in Oregon, Amy (The Tonic), Ana Burkham, Appleton King, Ben Wakeman, Bertus, Brooke Milde, Christine Wolf, Christy Cegelski, Chloe Hope, Colin & Gabriela, Corine Couturier, Dawn Kimble, Deborah T. Hewitt, Diana Freehill, Donna McArthur, E.T. Allen, Elissa Altman, Eleanor Anstruther, Elizabeth Hamilton, Eva Sikelianos, Gabe and Kristi Chikes, Gail Forrest, Gloria West, Grace Denali Dragonfly, Hannah Anstee, Heather Dupre, Heidi Piper, Holly Starley, James Warner, Jane Ratcliffe, Janet Ohanesian, Jan Cornell, Jen Cantwell, Jen Gatz, Jen Trepanier, Jeneye Abele, Jenna Newell Hiott, Jenny Jost, John Lovie, Joyce Wycoff, Julie Resnick, J.E. Moyer, Jan Cornell, Kate Mapother, Kathleen Waller, Kelly Pratt, Ken Riddle, Kevin Costello, Kristi Chikes, Laurie Michaels, Lili Lim, Linda Hoenigsberg, Lor, Luke Harold, Maddie Burton, Maria Popova, Maurice Clive Bisby, Mary Tabor, Michael Edward, Micah van Schalkwyk, Mr. Troy Ford, Mya Dexter, Nadia Gerassimenko, Nathan Slake, Nicola Corl, Nicole Foos, Patris, Paul Burnside, Patti Costello, Rex Wiig, Retta V, Rupal Rajani, Safar Fiertze, Sarah Copeland, Sarah Elizabeth, Sarah Fay, Satya Robyn, Shannon Kennedy, Shaler Wright, Soh-Yeon Lee, Susan Hamilton, Sydney, Tara Penry, Tanya Sanerib, Teyani Whitman, Theresa Taylor, Tim McLaughlin, Toni Prehoda Kahler, Veronika Bond. To bereavement groups like The Dougy Center—especially Jana DeCristofaro. To advocacy organizations: Health Story Collaborative, Global Genes, Vestibular Disorders Association, Life on the Level, Invisible Disabilities Association. To institutions that supported the long path here: Colorado College, National University of Natural Medicine, University of Wisconsin-Madison (to the kind librarian who found articles on

Charlie's disappearance—thank you). To my professional and social circles: Nikki Matthews and the entire Iridio team, Holly Gits, Martine Hammond, Robby Staley, Art Gallegos, Richard Lorimer, Julie Rood, Destiny Taylor, Maureen Burke, and the rest of my favorite photo team who held me when life's foundation cracked under me. And to friends of the past for shining your light on my path: Alejandro Plesch, Ana Burkham, Beau Young, Brooke Milde, Corinne Couturier, Greg Waters, Jenny Jost, Lauren Chandler, Linda Knittel, Paul VanGroll, Tamar Orlansky, Tanya Sanerib, Wendy Orth.

SPECIAL MENTIONS

To the entire Brauer and Breseman clans: your unwavering embrace taught me that family is sometimes a rediscovery. To the Warner-Palooza clan: thank you for seeing me whole—even in my shattered places—and for trusting that this memoir is, at its heart, a love story. And to the landscapes that shaped this book: the Midwestern soul rooted in kindness; Lake Michigan, keeper of Charlie's vanishing; Lake Winnebago, cradle of Dad's ashes—its waters flowing eastward, eventually joining the same vast lake, as if the two of them now drift together in one continuous, unseen current. Their waters, like their love, live on in me now.

If I forgot to name you, know that your impact still echoes. Your presence helped carry this story ashore.

TO OUR FOUNDERS

Every Empress Editions book is a declaration: midlife women are not a demographic—they're a cultural force.

This revolution wouldn't exist without the founding vision and bold support of **Shannon Kennedy** and **David Roberts**. They believed in our mission before the ink was dry and helped us build a publishing house devoted to amplifying the voices of women in their prime.

Shannon brings fierce heart and strategic clarity; David, sharp insight and unshakable belief. Together, they lit the match that started this fire.

To our founding visionaries: thank you for helping us turn the page on what publishing can be.

With gratitude and a glint of rebellion,

The Empress Editions Team

If you've enjoyed this Empress Editions book, why not write or telephone us for a free catalogue—or visit TheEmpressAge.com to join our Substack and discover more bold, midlife voices rewriting the rules.

Our authors love book clubs—especially the kind with mocktails and candor. Books ordered directly from Empress support a living legacy of matrilineal storytelling, healing, and cultural visibility.

Empress Editions
303 Third Street Cambridge, MA 02142
Telephone: +1 617.580.5266
hello@empresseditions.net
empresseditions.io

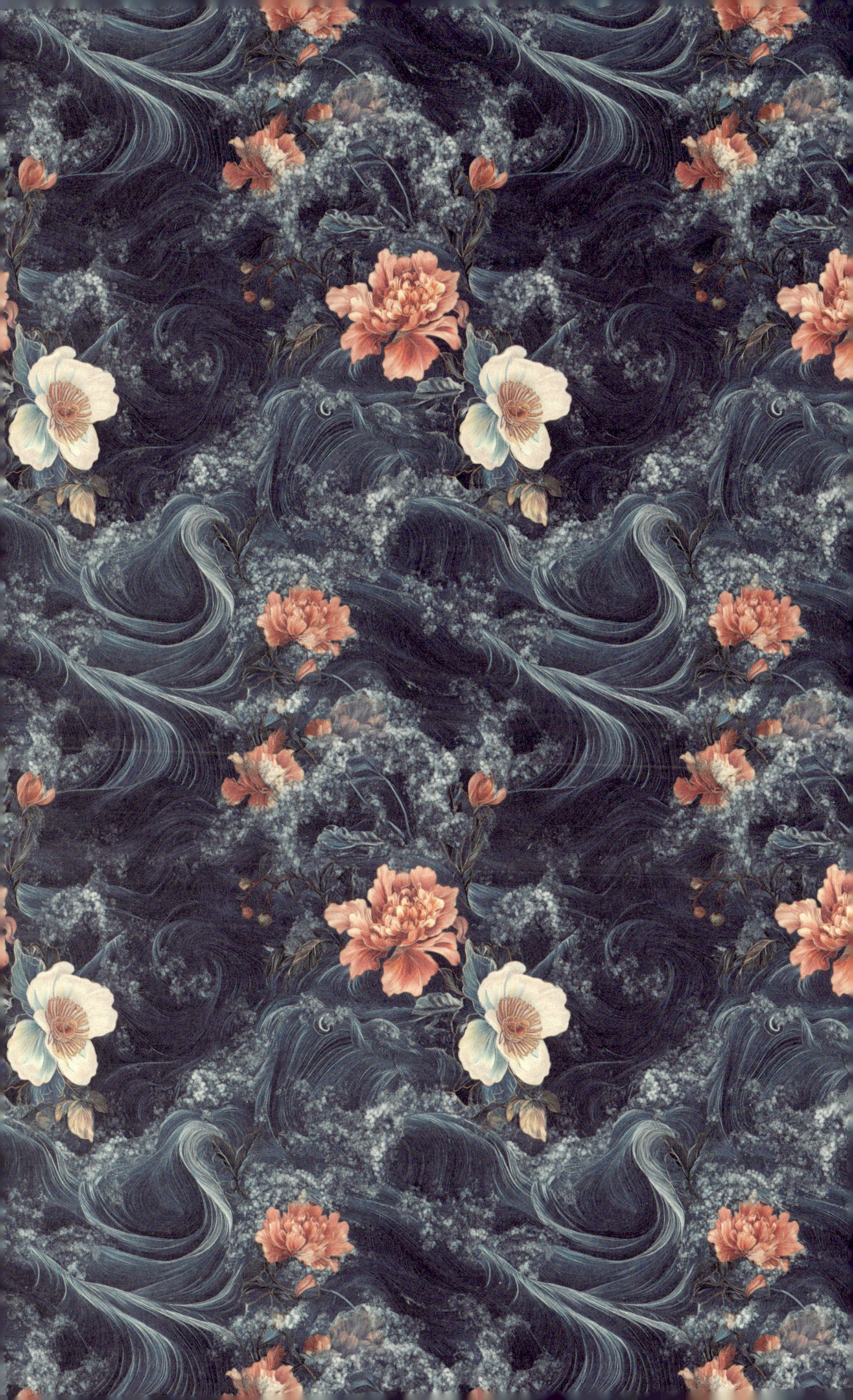

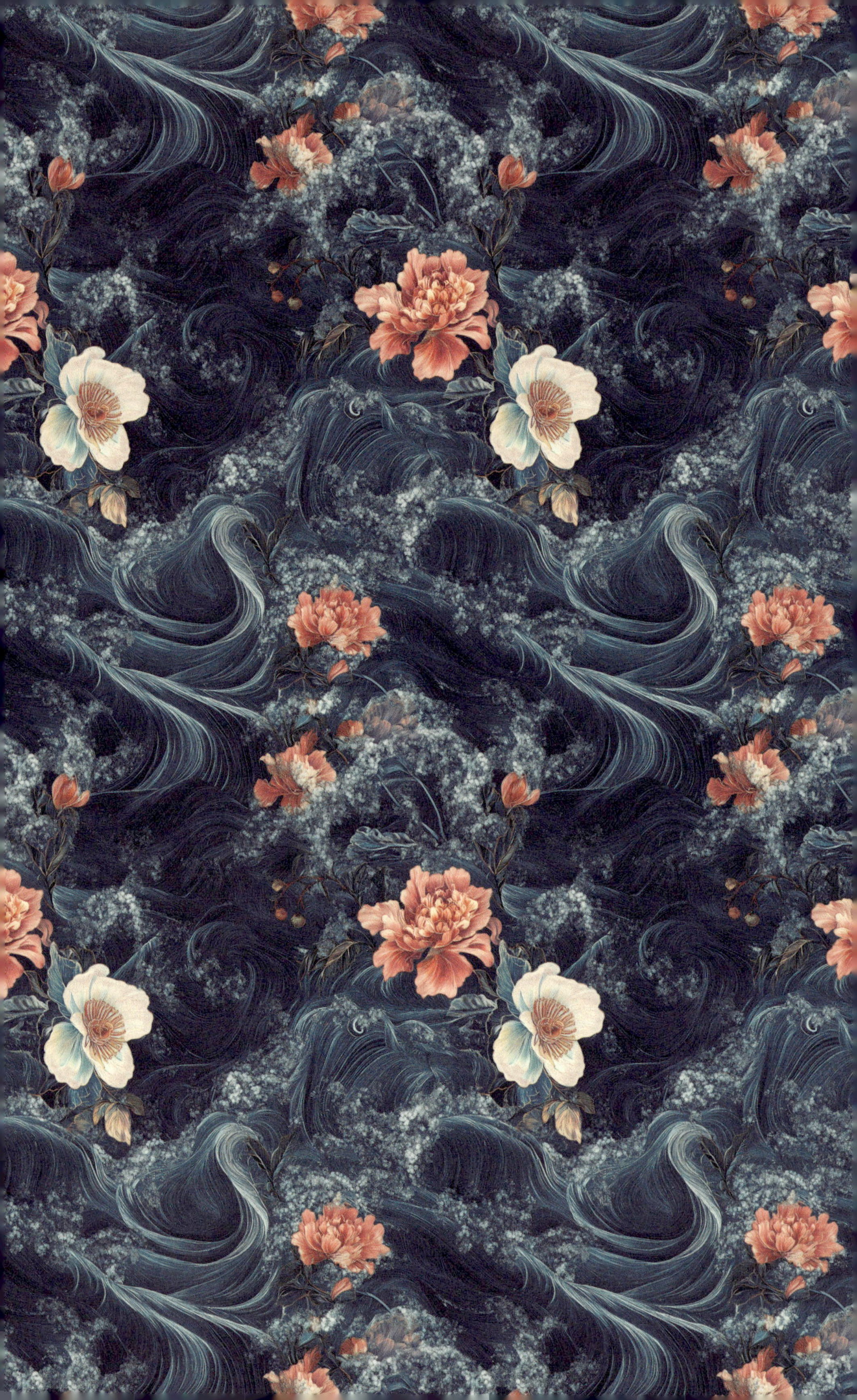